Real Life Heroes
Life Storybook

Real Life Heroes Life Storybook, 3rd Edition is a resourceful tool for children with traumatic stress. The resiliency-centered format and structure of the volume is coupled with treatment and sessions outlined in *Real Life Heroes: Toolkit for Treating Traumatic Stress in Children and Families*. This updated edition uses a creative arts approach, encouraging children to work with dependable adults to develop autobiographies through a wide range of activities, including drawings, music, movies, and narrative. By helping children feel protection from adversity and stressors that exist in everyday life, this workbook gives children a sense of value that can promote the transformation of troubled children from victims into tomorrow's heroes.

Richard Kagan, PhD, is the author and co-author of 10 books on treatment and services for children and families with traumatic stress and has published over 30 articles, chapters, and papers on practice and research issues in trauma therapy, child welfare, foster care, adoption, professional development, program evaluation, and quality improvement in family service and behavioral health care programs.

Real Life Heroes
Life Storybook

3rd Edition

Richard Kagan

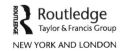

Routledge
Taylor & Francis Group

NEW YORK AND LONDON

Third edition published 2017
by Routledge
711 Third Avenue, New York, NY 10017

and by Routledge
2 Park Square, Milton Park, Abingdon, Oxon, OX14 4RN

Routledge is an imprint of the Taylor & Francis Group, an informa business

First edition published by Routledge 2004
Second edition published by Routledge 2007

Library of Congress Cataloging in Publication Data
A catalog record for this book has been requested

ISBN: 978-1-138-21784-3 (hbk)
ISBN: 978-0-415-51804-8 (pbk)
ISBN: 978-0-203-12356-0 (ebk)

Typeset in Times New Roman
by Florence Production Ltd, Stoodleigh, Devon, UK

Contents

Preface

Have you ever wondered what a real hero is like? I have.

"It's a person who will save you," one boy told me. Other boys and girls have told me how important it is to have people who care enough to tell the truth. A hero is "someone who you can look up to, someone you can depend on, someone who can help you," a teenage boy told me.

The dictionary says a hero is someone who is *the main character in a story*, someone *admired for his or her achievements and noble qualities*. A hero can be a *legendary figure known for great strength, ability, and courage*. We all know famous heroes from movies and books, and have learned about the courage of firefighters and police saving people and soldiers, sailors, and pilots fighting to protect people. I have also met boys and girls, moms and dads, grandparents, foster parents, teachers, and many others who have been real heroes, people who could be depended on to help, even if it meant taking great risks for their own lives.

I believe a hero can be a girl or a boy, a man or a woman. Most heroes do not ask to become known as heroes. Most heroes are regular people such as you or me with strengths and weaknesses, things that they are proud about and things they wish they had never done. What makes them heroes? I think heroes are people who keep on caring for others and helping others, even when they feel hurt, scared, lonely, or so mad they cannot think straight. Heroes keep going even when they know they have made mistakes and have their own problems. Heroes keep on caring and helping when times get tough.

It takes courage to be a hero, the courage to keep on going when you feel weak, the courage do the right thing when you could get in trouble. It also takes courage to learn new skills and to seek help for our own problems. Heroes help others and get help for themselves.

This is a book about using the skills and wisdom of heroes to get through 'tough times' and times that are so difficult that children and families get hurt in their bodies, their minds, and their most important relationships. This is a book for children, teenagers, parents, and other adults who care about children to learn new ways to make things better after 'tough times'.

You can use this book to look at the important people in your life, at home, at school, and in your neighborhood, and to find out who helped, who you could depend on, who told the truth, and who you could look up to as a hero. This is also a book about one special person: yourself. From the beginning to the end, it is all about you. You can even remove the *Real Life Heroes*® book cover and make up your own book cover, so this becomes your book from the front cover to the last page of the book.

I hope you will use this book to find what is special about yourself, your family, and the people who care about you, the special qualities that have helped you through good times and bad. When you do that, I think you will see that we can all be heroes in our own stories, the stories of our lives. And we don't have to do it alone.

Introduction for Parents and Caring Adults

Real Life Heroes Life Storybook, 3rd Edition is a workbook that helps children and adolescents develop self-esteem and overcome difficult experiences and traumas in their lives. The format helps children to create their own autobiographies with a wide range of activities, including drawings, photographs, music, dance, videotape, posters, crafts, and narrative. The workbook is designed for use by psychotherapists trained in trauma treatment. Parents, grandparents, teachers, foster parents, adoptive parents, and mentors can utilize the workbook with psychotherapists to help children develop increased resilience and reduce negative behaviors associated with a child's experiences of traumatic events, including losses, neglect, physical, sexual, or emotional abuse, domestic violence, community violence, wars, or natural disasters.

The workbook provides a tool for caring adults and psychotherapists to strengthen or rebuild ties to children and to foster well-being and security for children and their families. Therapists and counselors are urged to utilize *Real Life Heroes Toolkit* and *Rebuilding Attachments with Traumatized Children*, which include detailed guidelines on how to use this book for treatment of traumatic stress and Complex PTSD, including essential safety precautions, parenting tips, and a comprehensive guide to assessment and service planning for children with traumatic stress. The *Real Life Heroes Toolkit* provides a chapter-by-chapter reference, including:

- Objectives
- Overview
- Step by Step (key points and sequence)
- Pitfalls (problems that can undermine therapy)
- Strategies for overcoming challenges
- Checkpoints (essential elements)

The *Real Life Heroes Toolkit* includes tools to help parents, caring adults, and children understand and overcome traumas and to avoid re-traumatizing children by exposing them to reminders of the past or current stressful situations for which they are not prepared.

Drawings and storytelling are wonderful ways to help children foster a sense of mastery, positive values, and pride. By working together to share life experiences, caring adults can help children develop the courage and understanding they need to move beyond worries or fears from the past. Completing the *Real Life Heroes Life Storybook* provides a way for adults to show that they care enough about children to face difficult times and make things better.

Real Life Heroes® highlights and preserves moments in which important people in children's families and communities showed they cared, moments in children's lives that signify how they were valued. Parents and caring adults can use this book to show children that they can learn from the past, resolve problems in the present, and build a better future.

WHAT IS TRAUMATIC STRESS?

Children (and adults) can develop symptoms of traumatic stress when they experience events that threaten, or appear to threaten, severe harm, loss of emotionally supportive relationships, or death, and when a child or adult lacks the ability and supportive relationships to manage these threats. Experiences of natural disasters, deaths, severe illnesses, violence in the child's home or neighborhood, physical, sexual, or emotional abuse, and neglect can all lead to traumatic stress reactions. Traumatic events that affect a child's primary relationships can be especially harmful to a child's development.

When children feel their lives and the lives of those they love are no longer safe, they may develop long-lasting changes in how they think, feel, or respond with their bodies. Children's heart rates may increase and they may begin to sweat, become agitated, feel tense, feel aches or pains or 'butterflies in their stomachs,' and become hyper-alert. After a traumatic event, children may watch and listen vigilantly for signs that scary or dangerous things could happen again. Children may become emotionally upset with little warning and for reasons that are not noticed by other children or adults. They may also react by withdrawing, isolating, running away, getting into fights, or angrily lashing out at other children or adults. Repeated experiences of traumas can increase children's fears and behavioral reactions. Traumatic events that affect a child's primary relationships can be especially harmful to a child's development.

Traumatic stress reactions are often very distressing, but, in fact, these reactions are also very normal. These are ways our bodies protect us and prepare us to survive dangers. However, children who have experienced traumatic events may develop longer-lasting reactions that interfere with their physical and emotional health, especially if they have experienced multiple traumas that were unpredictable or disrupted children's relationships and security with caregivers. Children cannot learn or develop important social skills when they are always on the lookout for danger and when their bodies are ready to react quickly to any perception of risk for the child, family members, or other people children love. Attention and memory problems are common reactions, along with difficulty making plans or solving problems. Children with traumatic stress may fall behind in school and lack the ability to manage common requests by caregivers, teachers, or others in the community, leading to increased conflicts. Symptoms often include intense and ongoing emotional upset and agitation, chronic anxiety, behavioral changes, difficulties maintaining attention, school problems, nightmares, physical symptoms such as difficulty sleeping and eating, or symptoms of depression.

Traumatic stress may appear in different ways with different children. Reactions are often related to children's age, ability to understand, ability to cope, and feelings of security in their relationships with caregivers at the time that traumatic events occurred. One child in a family may react much more strongly than another child, often depending on their ability to cope and the support they experience during and after traumatic events. The good news is that treatments have been developed that can help children and their families who are suffering from traumatic stress.

HOW CAN LIFE STORY WORK HELP CHILDREN RECOVER AFTER TRAUMATIC EXPERIENCES?

Children often develop constricted beliefs and behaviors in order to cope with difficult times when they felt frightened, helpless, or even unwanted. A 12-year-old who lost his or her biological parents as a 4-year-old may continue to think and act very similarly to a preschooler. *Real Life Heroes*® helps parents and caring adults to nurture positive feelings of mastery, to overcome the hard times and any nightmares from the past, and to honor children's successes.

Life stories can help children develop confidence and self-respect. Life stories are especially important for children and parents who have experienced disruptions in primary relationships, the loss of important family members, or traumas. Hard times can be understood within the broader context of how family and community members acted to overcome problems. In this way, the past can be opened up from the perspective of strengths with stories of how the children were valued by parents, siblings, grandparents, aunts, uncles, cousins, foster parents, teachers, clergy, and other important people in their lives.

Life stories also provide a means of building a strong sense of family and cultural heritage. Fears and shame can be replaced by knowledge, insight, and the skills to cope with problems in the future. Beliefs centered on feelings of helplessness and weakness can be replaced by perceptions of how real people in each child's life have worked to make his or her life better. Working on a life story can change a child's perspective about his or her family's history and culture, and his or her present situation and opportunities. The life story approach helps children to capture stories of kindness, caring, and courage. Children learn how each of us makes a difference in our lives and in the lives of our families and communities.

Life stories and pictures can help children heal from past wounds without shaming them or running away from the truth. *Real Life Heroes*® provides activities in which caring adults can show children that they can deal with whatever the children have experienced, the good times and the bad. Life story work thus becomes a way for caring adults to rebuild or strengthen relationships based on nurture, protection, and commitment. These relationships, in turn, provide children with the foundations they need to develop empathy for others, to learn life skills, to take responsibility in their own lives, and to contribute to their communities.

Real Life Heroes® builds each child's sense of who has been a part of his or her life and who could help in the future. This is an activity for fostering a child's sense of him or herself as a hero with ties to family, friends, culture, and community.

A child's transformation from victim to hero requires safety, courage, and an ongoing relationship with a caring adult who values the child and sees his or her potential. Many children, very naturally, are afraid to face what they see as monsters from their past (or present). For a frightened child, this may be perceived as being asked to ford a raging river, impossible and terrifying. The child feels certain that he or she would be swept away.

Real Life Heroes® was created to help children step back from the river of their lives and to work with therapists and a parent or caring adult to build a sense of support from significant people in their past, the present, and for the future. Guided by committed and caring adults, children can find a place along the river where the water is still, shallow, and able to be crossed. Each story of support for the children and each example of how the children helped others forms a steppingstone for crossing the river. Together, these stories help children shape beliefs in themselves as heroes in their own lives.

HOW DOES REAL LIFE HEROES® WORK IN TREATMENT FOR TRAUMATIC STRESS?

Real Life Heroes® uses a *Life Storybook* and creative arts activities to help children and caregivers rebuild safety, caring, and resilience after experiences of traumatic stress. Workbook activities help children build the skills and security needed to foster healing, recovery, and the strength to overcome hardships. Children learn about what makes a hero, including learning skills to solve problems, getting help, and helping others. Learning about heroes includes learning about strengths and stories of how family members and people with the child's ethnic heritage have experienced and overcome hard times. Then, with these stories of caring and overcoming, children are encouraged to develop their own skills to succeed with help from caregivers.

In each session, children learn to recognize clues in their own bodies and how to share these safely with practitioners and caregivers. Sessions include sharing feelings on thermometers for stress, self-control, and feeling mad, sad, glad, and safe. Magic and calming activities engage children to learn and practice skills. Workbook pages help children share experiences and develop coping skills with rhythm, music, and movement. Therapists help children take their drawings and make them into short stories with a beginning, middle, and end so that children learn they can *move through* both good times, and later hard times, and make things better in their lives instead of feeling trapped.

Chapter by chapter, children work with caregivers and therapists to change cycles of behaviors that led to problems. Step-by-step activities help children grow stronger than their fears and to change old ways of coping that got them into more trouble. The workbook helps children change how they see themselves from feeling hurt, unwanted, unlikeable, damaged, or hopeless, to feeling that they can work through the traumas of the past to experiences of safety with caring adults committed to helping children grow and develop into adulthood.

Real Life Heroes® helps children develop hope, skills, and confidence with the support of caring adults. The *Life Storybook* highlights each child's and family's strengths, including their spiritual and cultural heritage, and provides activities that practitioners and caregivers can use to help each child grow strong enough to change problems. Each chapter develops skills and relationships needed for the next chapter, leading up to helping the child reduce traumatic stress reactions. The model works like a pyramid for growth, step by step, chapter by chapter.

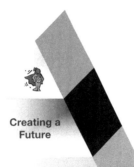

Creating a
Future

Developing a Life Story
of Overcoming

*Moving Through the
Tough Times* Instead of
Re-living the Past

**Developing the Hero Inside;
Coping and Survival Skills**

**Strengthening Emotionally Supportive
& Enduring Relationships;** *Allies,
Mentors, & Guardians*

**Rebuilding Security and Co-regulation with
Caring Adults; Creative Arts & Life Stories**

**Developing Self-regulation and Safety Skills
Inspired by Heroes;** *Power Plans*

Learning *to Recognize, Express and Modulate Feelings;
SOS for Stress*

Real Life Heroes® is listed in the National Registry of Evidence-Based Programs and Practices by the Substance Abuse Mental Health Services Administration (SAMHSA), the SAMHSA National Center for Trauma-Informed Care "Models for Developing Trauma-Informed Behavioral Health Systems and Trauma-Specific Services," and as one of the National Child Traumatic Stress Network's (NCTSN) Empirically Supported Treatments and Promising Practices.

HOW ARE PAGES OF THE *LIFE STORYBOOK* USED?

On each page of the workbook, a caption (instruction) is printed at the top, with space below for a drawing, a photograph, or a representation of what the children demonstrated. Lines at the bottom can be used to write in a story of what was remembered, as well as images, a poem, or songs that the children remember. *Real Life Heroes®* was especially written for children between the ages of 6 and 12, but can easily be adapted for adolescents by using the themes addressed on each page and creative approaches outlined in the *Real Life Heroes Toolkit*. The *Real Life Heroes Toolkit* also includes guidelines to adapt the book for use with younger children. Word processing programs can be used to create stories that can be pasted into the book or printed directly on the bottom of photocopied pages under pictures. Or, audiotapes or videotapes could be made to accompany the pictures, page by page.

Real Life Heroes® can be tailored to best help each child. Therapists and parents can use or omit pages to match each child's special situation and can duplicate pages as needed to enrich an important story in each child's life. The most important pages are marked by a superhero figure:

The heading at the top of the page directs children to think about a memory or a fantasy and then picture it in a space below with a drawing or a photograph, imagine how it would sound as a drumbeat or a song, and show how it would look through movement as a dance or movie. It helps to ask the child to do these steps without any words. After the child draws a picture and shares it with rhythm, music, and movement, safe, caring adults repeat the rhythm, music, and movement shared by children to promote emotional attunement and strengthen relationships with caregivers after traumatic experiences. This is outlined in the *Real Life Heroes Toolkit* and described in more detail below. The question at the bottom of the page can be used to direct children to use words to write a brief note about something special in their picture. Questions were designed to build up children's sense of being valued and their sense of competence in different situations. The completed page will typically contain both children's visual memories and a short narrative to add additional details and their understanding of what was most important.

WHAT'S INSIDE EACH CHAPTER?

The *Life Storybook* works progressively to build the child's self-regulation skills, trust in relationships, and to reduce the impact of traumatic stress. When safe caregivers are involved, the *Life Storybook* and *Real Life Heroes®* activities also promote development of co-regulation that can be maintained in families. Chapter 1 provides an introduction to how stress from 'tough times' and traumatic events can lead to traumatic stress and, conversely, how building skills for modulation and strengthening emotionally supportive relationships can help children stay in control, prevent, or heal, from traumatic stress, and achieve their goals. Chapter 1 encourages children to develop initial safety plans and *Pocket Power Cards* that can help remind of them of how they can reduce stress and traumatic stress reactions.

In Chapter 2, children are invited to share a little about themselves with counselors and caregivers who are helping them write this book, and by so doing, to see that it is normal to have a wide range of feelings. This is especially important for children who have experienced separations and traumas leading them to become constricted in their feelings, beliefs, and skills and to lack hope for change. Traumatized children also often develop constricted abilities to understand the feelings shown by adults and peers and then react to their misperceptions of people around them. Chapter 2 helps children learn to more accurately recognize feelings of adults and other children in their families, schools, and communities, and to express their own feelings in appropriate ways. Parents and other adults can use this chapter to show children how they see them as special and that they are committed to listening to them and respecting their perspectives. Chapter 2 gives adults an opportunity to validate how children have been successful and to show acceptance of their wide range of feelings. Children who feel they can trust the adults who are helping them will be much more willing to move ahead in the book.

The heroes theme promotes hope that children and the adults who care about children can make things better and encourages children to learn skills modeled by the people and fictional characters they admire. Chapter 3 builds on the conception of heroes as people who help others and contribute to their families and communities. Helping others is an integral part of building self-esteem and shaping tomorrow's citizens and leaders. In Chapter 3, children are invited to draw, act out, or write brief stories of people in their lives who acted like a hero. By making this a shared activity with a parent, relative, or committed adult, children learn that they are not alone and that important people in their lives can see the importance of caring for one another. At the same time, adults can learn from children what they look for in a hero. Chapter 3 also provides a place for children to remember how they have helped others and to envision what they could do in the future to help make things better for their families and communities.

Chapter 3 emphasizes the courage to help others and the making of a hero, including the power of self-awareness, self-soothing, and focusing skills as common attributes of heroes. Chapter 4 builds on the image of heroes to help children develop their own self-awareness of strengths, stressors, typical reactions, and ways they can make things better with help from caring adults. These are skills that children can develop with practice, including exercises in therapy sessions and 'homework' assignments. Development of abilities to self-monitor, relax, and refocus are outlined in detail in the *Real Life Heroes Toolkit*. Chapter 4 helps children put this together into a detailed safety plan that can be condensed into a *Pocket Power Card* for children to carry with them. Caregivers can complete their own Power Plan, which is provided separately in the *Real Life Heroes Toolkit*.

Chapter 5 helps children to remember people who cared for them, day to day, through sickness and health. Memories of being valued and of positive people are often lost or minimized when a child has experienced difficult times. This chapter provides an opportunity to expand children's awareness of people who have helped, even in small ways, and to highlight resources in their lives, including their own talents. Children can also be encouraged to share (and discover) images of heroes from their family's heritage, stories of family members triumphing over adversity, rituals, and richness in the family's cultural background. Chapter 5 encourages children to learn about family stories passed on from generation to generation, favorite music, family photos and movies, and the hopes, wishes, wisdom, and special accomplishments of previous generations. This chapter also includes a template to help children diagram the roots of their family tree, highlighting ties to family members, friends, caring adults, and levels of support.

Chapter 6 helps children to remember and record the strengths, skills, and supportive relationships that helped them in 'good times.' Children can then utilize these memories and counselors or therapists can bring in safe supportive adults to help them to learn from their 'tough times'.

Chapter 7 invites children to make things better in their lives, working from magical wishes and reinforcing work on developing self-soothing and mindfulness skills. Therapists and caring adults can assess whether a child is ready to move on to more difficult issues by children's demonstration of the ability to relax themselves and manage stress with the help of safe caregivers.

Chapter 8 helps children learn the power of shaping their beliefs, changing from catastrophic thinking to courageous thinking, and challenges children to defeat traumas by developing skills. This chapter includes an introduction to how traumatic stress builds on painful experiences, negative thinking, and common reactions that lead to even more trouble, 'tough times', and often self-denigration. Chapter 8 stresses how children can grow stronger by changing their life stories, working step by step to change how they understand and react to problems.

Chapter 9 provides a chronicle for a child's moves between different locations or homes. Children can also use this section to develop a timeline of good and bad events. Ratings of events from 'worst' to 'best' can help children to see how forces outside their control have affected their lives *and* at the same time to develop a sense of time, including a past, a present, and a future. This helps children develop the understanding that they don't have to remain stuck in an uncomfortable position.

After a child completes the timeline, it is helpful to emphasize how we can learn from the bad times, but it is even more important to learn from the good times. Ask the child to draw a line connecting each circled number on the right side. Then, turn the page horizontally so the page number is on the right side. It helps to highlight every year in the child's life when the line went up and to discuss with the child how these were some of the times in his or her life when things got better. The child can be asked to think about who helped in these special times and how the child helped him or herself.

The timeline helps to identify positive events and upswings in children's lives. By looking more closely at these important and often neglected times, caring adults can help children learn lessons about important people who helped them succeed, how they helped themselves, and how they and important people in their lives overcame problems. In this way, successes from the past can expand a child's sense of hope to deal with problems in the present or the future.

Chapter 10 provides an opportunity for therapists to help children re-experience progressively more difficult 'tough times' in a safe way, building on children's expanded understanding, skills, and ability to call upon help from caring adults, mentors, and friends. Use of creative arts modalities (see *Real Life Heroes Toolkit*) helps children reduce the pain associated with 'tough times' while building new and more constructive beliefs, stories, and skills for overcoming difficulties. The chapter concludes with an opportunity for children to think about what they could do to make up for mistakes they have made.

Chapter 11 provides a chance for children to develop images of themselves becoming successful in the future. This can easily lead to planning activities and educational programs to help children achieve their goals. As with earlier chapters, Chapter 11 highlights the importance of safe relationships with people who can help children.

By the end of this book, children should be able to identify people who cared about them in the past and the present, and who they'd like to have in their lives in the future. Children should also be able to verbalize, picture, or dramatize what they have learned about themselves and their families.

In Chapter 12, children are invited to create their own title page as the final step in this book with a title that reflects how they have mastered 'good times and bad.' Examples of titles include: "My Book about Good Times and Bad," "All about Me," "My Family and Me," "My Life from A to Z," and "How I Learned to Enjoy My Life." Children are then encouraged to either replace the original book cover with their own title page or, if they wish, to remove the original book cover, introduction for adults, the 'About the Author' page, and any unused pages. This makes the book entirely their own work.

Chapter contents are listed in the box below as a reference.

CHAPTER CONTENTS

Chapter 1: The Heroes Challenge

- Children and caregivers read about how stress can build up inside our brains and our bodies to the point that we feel out of control.

- Workbook pages show children how they can build self-control power and relationships to help them grow stronger and reduce traumatic stress.

Chapter 2: A Little About Me

- Children (and caregivers) begin to use workbook pages to develop stories with feelings expressed through rhythm, music, and movement.

- Chapter pages encourage children to develop skills and safety to recognize a range of feelings, express feelings appropriately, and change how they feel so they can remain safe.

Chapter 3: Heroes

- Children identify heroes they see in media, popular culture, politics, their cultural heritage, and their family, and learn what helps their heroes succeed, including how heroes get help and help others.

- Workbook pages encourage children and caregivers to share stories of overcoming 'tough times' by family members and highlight the importance of caregivers for helping children learn essential skills and developing courage.

Chapter 4: Power Plans

- Children build on their awareness of how heroes use skills to look at what has helped them, 'tough times' in their lives, typical reactions to stress, and how they can use skills and support from safe caregivers and other caring adults to make things better.

- Children develop *Youth Power Plans*, strength-based worksheets that focus on helping children share what helps them cope, what doesn't help, and developing a shared safety plan with caring adults to prevent or reduce traumatic stress reactions.

- Caregivers are also encouraged to develop *Caregiver Power Plans* that identify their child's triggers, reactions, and interventions that can prevent or reduce traumatic stress reactions.

- *Power Plans* are condensed into *Pocket Power Cards* that children can carry with them.

Chapter 5: My Family

- Children and caregivers work together as detectives to learn about who helped children in the past and to record memories of caring.

- Children's skills and talents are linked with achievement of parents, grandparents, other relatives, and stories of overcoming that are part of children's cultural heritage.

Chapter 6: Important People

- Children (and caregivers) explore a broad range of people in their lives and identify mentors, protectors, and emotionally supportive relationships.

- Memories of support are strengthened to expand the child's sense of security and confidence.

Chapter 7: Mind Power

- Children develop resources within themselves and with the help of supportive adults to calm down through slow breathing, reminders of caring, comforting images, positive beliefs, focusing their attention, and movement.

- Activities strengthen skills for self-regulation by developing the child's ability to become aware of signals in his or her body, how feelings and thoughts can come and go, how the child can redirect attention, and open up possibilities for making things better.

- Children develop skills that help them accept and move through fears and negative thoughts and try out new behaviors to solve problems.

- Children increase development of skills to manage situations that can often trigger traumatic stress reactions, including how to stay safe in relationships, develop positive friendships, and learn from teachers, coaches, clergy, and other safe and supportive adults.

Chapter 8: Changing the Story

- Worksheet questions help children recognize how stress works in the body and mind and how changing beliefs about themselves can help the children achieve their goals and make things better for themselves and their families.

- Children are invited to become the directors of their own 'life' movies as a way to engage them to take control of what happens when they are triggered with reminders that have, in the past, led to problem behaviors.

- Activities include breaking apart what happens leading to distress and getting into trouble, and how children can become 'thought-shifters' to succeed.

- Working on this chapter with supportive caregivers helps children feel safe enough to share how they felt and acted in the past and how they can feel safe again with caring adults committed to protecting and guiding the child to maturity.

Chapter 9: Looking Back

- A roadmap and timeline help children remember important people and places from the past and to organize what happened in their lives by the years of their lives, from birth to the present time.

- Chapter pages encourage children to share how they remember places where they lived, the people who cared for them, how they felt in each place, and how they experienced and understood what led to them moving to a new home now that they are older (and wiser).

- Chapter 9 helps caregivers and practitioners understand the child's experiences (feelings and beliefs) and develop a list of traumatic events to help the child reintegrate traumatic experiences with a renewed sense of safety.

Chapter 10: Through the 'Tough Times'

- Workbook pages help children and emotionally supportive caregivers to safely share what they experienced in stressful events, what was most difficult, and what they learned can make things better.

- Movies and 'Five-Chapter' Stories help children share traumatic experiences, stressing how the children and supportive adults have developed skills and supports so they can escape feeling trapped in recurrent traumatic experiences.

- Activities encourage use of evidence-supported desensitization techniques to help children feel safe and supported enough to share undisclosed details and 'move through' traumatic memories with emotional support from therapists and caregivers and with use of their Mind Power skills to places and times where they felt safe and cared for.

- Children are encouraged to share any experiences of loss and also any shame for what they feel they have done wrong and to find ways to feel good about themselves again.

- Before completing Chapter 8, practitioners and caregivers help children practice 'moving through' their worst memories with emotional support from therapists and caregivers and with use of their Mind Power skills so that reminders of what happened and other hard times will not lead to traumatic stress reactions.

Chapter 11: Into the Future

- Workbook pages encourage children to broaden their sense of time by sharing how they see themselves developing skills and relationships through adolescence and into adulthood.

- Activities encourage children to share who they would see as important in their lives and provide opportunities for practitioners and caregivers to build or strengthen positive, supportive relationships with family members, mentors, and other supportive adults.

> **Chapter 12: My Story**
>
> - 'My Story' provides an opportunity for children to integrate what they have learned into life stories of overcoming shared in words with photos, drawings, or video.
>
> - Children are invited to share what they have learned and how they would help other children who experienced similar 'tough times' as they did, building children's sense of themselves as heroes helping others.
>
> - Children are then urged to cut off the *Real Life Heroes®* book cover and substitute their own book cover and dedication to make this book truly their own.

SAFETY FIRST

Children need to feel protected by the adults who are raising them and safe from any threats of violence, emotional abuse, neglect, or other forms of intimidation. Children should never be asked to share feelings or memories with adults with whom they do not feel emotionally and physically safe. The *Real Life Heroes Toolkit* outlines safety criteria for involving adults in life story work and other activities. Safety criteria includes adults showing a commitment to keeping children safe from emotional, physical, or sexual abuse, validating children's feelings and experiences, and working, to help children (and families) heal from past traumas and prevent recurrence of traumatic events. Children also need to have developed skills in calming themselves before completing Chapter 10 in order to avoid rekindling and strengthening trauma reactions. The *Real Life Heroes Toolkit* (see Resource Checklist in Part V) provides a checklist of essential skills and resources needed *before* encouraging children to re-experience past traumas.

Children must feel free to be able to signal or say, "Stop, I need to take a break," and then be able to utilize some form of distraction, imagery, tension release, physical exercise, prayer, or meditation to soothe themselves. Therapists and teachers using this workbook need to be able to work individually with each child and ensure confidentiality as needed.

Remembering past events can rekindle both happy and painful feelings, including sadness, loneliness, or anger. This is a natural part of healing. To make this process more understandable, it is helpful to point out to children that these feelings are normal and that it is natural for them to sometimes remember other events later on. This can be presented as a natural process in developing strength and mastering old problems.

It is important for the adults involved to help a child relax and feel safe. Knowing the child involved is essential. A hug from a trusted family member, a pat on the back, and praise for the child's courage may be all that is needed. For other children, extended practice in relaxation techniques and reduction of feelings of shame with help from a therapist may be needed.

If children have experienced traumas, appear agitated, lose awareness of what is happening around them, or act in ways that put themselves or others at risk of being hurt, writing this book should be guided by a skilled trauma therapist (licensed psychologists, social workers, or psychiatrists), who can provide a comprehensive assessment of the child within the family and help parents and children work together. Children showing signs of acute stress often need help to feel safe at home, at school, or in their neighborhoods. The *Real Life Heroes Toolkit* provides guidelines for assessing children's feelings of safety in relationships and developing safety plans.

Tension or distress in children often reflects very normal reactions to real crises. Children's behaviors, the words they use, and the feelings they show can guide caring adults to old problems or previous traumas that still bother children. Assessment tools provided in the *Real Life Heroes Toolkit* and other standardized measures of trauma and psychological functioning can be used to help therapists and caregivers understand what is driving traumatic stress reactions and identify clues from children about what could help them to develop more effective coping strategies. Therapists, parents, and other caring adults can then help children to overcome specific fears and memories of events that shaped their lives.

ATTUNEMENT AND VALIDATION

Real Life Heroes® works best as a shared activity guided by a psychologist, social worker, or psychiatrist, along with the primary adult or adults who are working to provide children with safe, nurturing homes, adults who children can trust to believe and protect them. The *Real Life Heroes Toolkit* outlines how safe, caring adults can complete pages of the work along with children including expressing feelings and meaning for each page in rhythm, tonality and movement. Caring adults can also mirror their child's rhythm, tonality, and movement expressed for each picture drawn by the child. This promotes literal attunement between children and caregivers to strengthen emotionally supportive relationships and build, or rebuild, trust that children can share feelings with caregivers. Children can also be asked to mirror adults' rhythm, tonality, and movement for adults' pictures to reinforce connections and help caregivers model what has helped them and how they manage stressful situations.

The success of these activities relies largely on the ability of the adults in children's lives to show that children will truly be safe to share. For children, this means that the adults involved will validate their experiences and feelings and will help them to overcome distressing and shameful problems. This begins with a pledge at the beginning of the book for adults to show that they want children to share what they think, remember, and feel.

Children cannot be expected to work on life stories if they are being asked to deny their experiences or to return to a home or school marked by threats, emotional abuse, or violence. Similarly, children cannot be expected to utilize life stories for positive growth if the adults around them do not have the courage to speak honestly about what has happened and to take responsibility for their own actions. Children learn to deal with the truth from their parents and significant adults in their lives.

Caring adults and counselors need to respect children's natural feelings of loyalty to parents, relatives, and other adults (foster parents, teachers, mentors) who have acted as primary caregivers to them in the past. Subtle or overt pressure by family members or other adults to say or 'remember' certain events in a certain way, positive or negative, will lead to greater constriction in children and will often generate misunderstandings and accelerate behavior problems. If children show any signs of feeling pressured to say or remember in a way to please family members, foster parents, or other significant people, it is essential to have a neutral therapist to guide this work and work with family members and any service providers to keep the children safe. If family members or other adults contradict children and tell them they are wrong, therapists can meet the children alone and ask them how they experienced the event in question, validating the children's own memories. Then, the therapist can ask the children what they thought and felt about the adult who told the children they were wrong. In some cases, this may represent two different perceptions. In other cases, the children may be experiencing pressure to remember events in the way a family member wants instead of how the children actually perceived what happened. If children are intimidated in any way, or frightened by an adult's invalidation, it would be important to stop any conjoint life story work with that adult until the adult can develop the capacity to validate the children's perceptions.

Most children will test adults quickly to see if adults will believe them. Caring adults need to know that this process of testing is both normal and necessary for children to find out if it is safe to open up their feelings and beliefs. Children need to find out if adults will criticize them in a shaming manner or become too stressed to deal with real situations and experiences. Validation can be facilitated by allowing young children to dictate to adults. Adults can help by carefully writing down what the children say, using their words. Children can then see that the adults are truly hearing their stories and not trying to change them to fit the adult's perspective or wishes.

This should not become a forced project for children to work on by themselves, although some children may prefer to do sections by themselves and then share these parts later. And, some children may not have caregivers they can fully trust. The *Real Life Heroes Toolkit* outlines how counselors and therapists can help these children and their families. Ideally, caring adults work on their own life stories at the same time or ahead of children. Caring adults involved in treatment are asked to complete their own copy of the *Real Life Heroes Life Storybook* or write their own story as a narrative in a way that children can understand in an age-appropriate manner that will not push children beyond their capacity to manage stress. Caring adults are also asked to highlight how they would handle the different questions raised in each of the 12 chapters of this workbook and and show how they have developed the awareness, skills, and capacity to reinforce 'good times' and to validate and manage 'tough times' while protecting themselves and their families. In this way, caring adults can demonstrate that it is OK to share both good and bad memories without shame or embarrassment. Caring adults can also pass on what they learned in their own lives, and in particular, how they learned to get the help they needed and to help others. If a parent is too uncomfortable to work together with their child on sharing their experiences, it is often helpful to bring in a trusted relative, mentor or friend who will validate the child and who may be more comfortable sharing feelings and can support the child and caregiver in addition to a therapist.

ENHANCING CREATIVITY

There are no right or wrong stories and no right or wrong ways to share feelings and memories. Some children are better with words. Some prefer visual images, music, or movement to show how they feel and understand situations. Children's creative strengths facilitate resolution of conflicts in ways that would be impossible if they were required to work within one framework, such as verbally telling what happened. Moreover, painful memories are stored at different levels and associated with different senses such as visual images, touch, smell, auditory memory, or feelings.

Children are invited at the end of Chapter 2 to share photographs or drawings of themselves showing different feelings. For children who have difficulty recognizing or expressing different feelings, it often helps to practice identifying and expressing differ-ent feelings. Fears, inhibitions, and traumas may lead children to become constricted in their abilities to express basic feelings. Use of pictorial charts of different feelings can provide a reference and looking at photographs from magazines can be used to practice understanding other people's expressions. A video camera, digital camera, or instant camera can provide a fun means to practice expressing feelings. Such exercises can be used to show children that it is normal and expected for them to show a wide range of feelings. Adults could also model how they can show different feelings in their faces, tone of voice, words, and actions. For children with an aptitude for physical expression, this can be enlarged into activities to express emotions and messages through move-ment and dance. Growth and recovery from trauma are fostered by having a child develop creative and flexible responses. It helps to begin this process in Chapter 1 and then to continue this for each chapter by asking the child, for each page, to draw (or photograph) an image, accentuate facial details, tap out a rhythm and intensity to match the child's drawing, add tones from a simple xylophone or other musical instrument, and then to enact what they represented as a movement, dance, or a sports move tied with feelings shown in their pictures (e.g., a 'happy' dunk shot in basketball, or a 'sad' free shot, a 'powerful' 'bended' soccer kick at the goal). Children can then be asked to identify feelings expressed in their drawings with words, to highlight posi-tive beliefs stressing strengths and coping strategies, to reinforce getting help from safe adults or peers, including family members, mentors, teachers, and friends, and helping others.

Children can choose between creative approaches such as drawings, posters, stories, poetry, music, videotapes, collages of pictures cut from magazines or picture books, cartoons, interviews with adults in the format of news shows, dance or movement patterns recorded on videotape, 'improv' activities, or other creative approaches that tap into their special talents. Photographs could also be collected (or copied) from relatives and inserted along with other important documents. It helps to have a smartphone or camera that can generate immediate digital images and be used to print photographs in a timely manner. It also helps to begin this work by giving children a special set of markers or colored pencils reserved for work on the *Life Storybook*.

STORYTELLING

Children learn to love reading books with a parent, teacher, or another caring person who sits with them, repeats their beloved stories, and later guides them at their pace to start reading themselves. Similarly, storytelling may be facilitated when safe caring adults work closely with children. Sitting close and forms of guidance should match each child's level of comfort and the child's emotional and developmental age. For example, a 10-year-old who feels and acts as a 5-year-old may need the same level of nurture and assistance as a 5-year-old in order to overcome past traumas.

Adults can help children to develop each story by gently asking them to write or share what they remember and to make up a brief story to go along with the picture. For younger or more hesitant children, the adult can write out the children's dictated stories on notepaper or on a word processor. Then, either the adult or the children can copy or paste the story onto the appropriate page of the *Real Life Heroes Life Storybook*.

Maintaining a backup copy of the *Life Storybook* in a safe place is highly recommended and therapists are encouraged to keep the *Life Storybook* in their offices until completion. After completing the book, children may wish to put it aside. It helps to laminate the finished book to show that it is special and something the children may want to look at again when they are 5, 10, or 20 years older, just like a time capsule. A parent can offer to keep the book in a safe place, to be read again whenever children wish.

STRENGTHENING RELATIONSHIPS, BUILDING SELF-ESTEEM

Children learn to see themselves by how important people in their lives demonstrate they care in good times and bad. Children who have experienced emotional, physical or sexual abuse, multiple separations or other relational traumas may show little trust in themselves or anyone else. Even a sense of hope may be lacking. And caregivers may feel they have lost positive relationships with children after going through hard times. The *Life Storybook* can be used in attachment-centered trauma treatment to help rebuild attachments, a critical component in helping children overcome the impact of multiple traumas.

As noted above, parents and other caring adults can be included in work on *Real Life Heroes®* pages if they meet safety criteria outlined in the *Real Life Heroes Toolkit*. This helps to strengthen (or build) child-caregiver relationships and to heal gaps that may have developed when children and adults experienced traumatic events.

When caregivers are included in sessions, it helps to have adults complete their own responses to workbook pages and then to share their own experiences in a way that helps pass on what they have learned. As noted above, sharing needs to be done at a level that children can handle at their point of social, emotional, and cognitive development. Sharing also needs to be limited to what children can manage without overwhelming them with adult fears. A therapist can guide sessions to help caregivers model how to move through hard times and how caring adults have made their families and communities safe so children no longer have to fear repetition of traumatic events.

Rebuilding relationships takes courage, time, and effort. This book was developed to help parents and other caring adults to nurture positive feelings of mastery, to overcome fears, and to honor children's and caregivers' successes. Their completed books represent a testament to children's courage and the adults who worked with them to maintain (or rekindle) hope. Children's life storybooks can become a symbol of how children and emotionally supportive caregivers have become stronger together than the nightmares of the past.

About the Author

Dr. Kagan provides consultation and training on traumatic stress and complex trauma treatment including *Real Life Heroes®* certificate training programs. He has had extensive leadership experience in non-profit child and family services as director of professional development, QI, research, and psychological services and has served as the principal investigator for two SAMHSA-funded National Child Traumatic Stress Network (NCTSN) community practice site grants. Dr. Kagan has also served on the NCTSN Steering Committee, the NCTSN Affiliate Advisory Board, the Complex Trauma and Child Welfare Committees, and co-led development of the NCTSN curriculum, *Caring for Children Who Have Experienced Traumatic Stress*. He was formerly Director of Research and Consultation for the Sidney Albert Training and Research Institute at Parsons Child and Family Center in Albany, New York, a NCTSN community services site since 2002.

Dr. Kagan is the author and co-author of ten books: *Families in Perpetual Crisis* with Shirley Schlosberg (Norton); *Turmoil to Turning Points: Building Hope for Children in Crisis Placements* (Norton); *Wounded Angels: Lessons from Children in Crisis* (Child Welfare League of America); *Wounded Angels: Inspiration from Children in Crisis* (Routledge); *Rebuilding Attachments with Traumatized Children: Healing from Losses, Violence, Abuse, and Neglect* (Routledge); *Real Life Heroes: A Life Storybook for Children,* 1st, 2nd and 3rd Editions (Routledge); *Real Life Heroes Practitioner's Manual* (Routledge); and *Real Life Heroes Toolkit for Treating Traumatic Stress in Children and Families* (Routledge). He has published over 30 articles, chapters, and papers on practice and research issues in trauma therapy, child welfare, foster care, adoption, professional development, program evaluation, and quality improvement in family service agencies. Dr. Kagan's presentations, articles, and books highlight practical and innovative approaches that practitioners and organizations can utilize to help children and families strengthen resilience and reduce traumatic stress. Further information about Dr. Kagan's publications and training programs can be found at www.reallifeheroes.net.

The Pledge

It is important to work on this book with someone you can trust to help you and keep you safe. Before sharing a little about yourself, please ask any adults who are helping you to sign below.

"I promise to help _____ [name of youth] in any way I can. This is his or her book and I want him or her to use it to share whatever he or she thinks, remembers, and feels."

_____   _____

_____   _____

_____   _____

_____   _____

[name]   [date]

[If any adults join you later to help, please be sure to ask them to sign this page first.]

Chapter 1

The Heroes Challenge

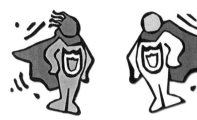

'Tough times' start the alarm[1] bells ringing in our bodies. It may be scary, it may hurt, but it also helps. We feel our stomachs get tighter, our hearts beating faster, our arms and legs get ready for action. These are like little *Knots*[2] that wake us up to start thinking and do something to solve a problem.

Power for heroes means using our whole selves, our whole bodies from the tips of our toes to the thinking power of our brains. Power means self awareness and self control, the ability to use our strengths and skills to reach our goals, like a pilot steering a jet plane to reach a distant city and then making a safe landing on the runway of the airport, not too fast, not too slow. We can call this *Self-Control Power* because it's ours, but only if we want to own it and use it. *Self-Control Power* is a skill, just like learning to ride a bike or shoot a basket, a skill we can grow stronger and stronger, stronger than the alarm bells that warn us of danger.

Every day, every year, we can grow our *Self-Control Power* and become stronger and smarter. Children learn to take control of their bodies and make things better from the time they are born. Babies cry and someone who cares for the child, a mother, a father, a grandpa, a grandma, comes and makes them feel better. The caring adult calms the child down. Later, as the child grows bigger, caring adults and children learn to calm down together. That's called 'co-regulation,' a big word that really means something very simple: adults who care about a child can help that child stay safe and feel better in 'tough times'. And, when the child grows bigger, the child learns to calm down by him or herself. That's called 'self-control.' But, the truth is, no matter whether you are 2 years old, 22, or 62, 'people need people.' Girls and boys, mothers and fathers, grandparents, aunts, uncles, teachers, police officers, even presidents, need other people. It's just the way it is.

Self-Control Power also means knowing everyone gets worried sometimes. Worries and fears are natural. They give us energy. With *Self-Control Power*, we can think and plan and solve problems. And, we can get help from safe, caring adults and friends. With *Self-Control Power*, we can help ourselves and the people we care about.

But, sometimes the 'tough times' are so horrible that our stomachs may start to ache. Our hearts feel like drums beating faster and faster until they feel like they might explode, and our arms and legs feel so tight they may burn. We may feel stuck, helpless, no good, or terrified. Things may seem especially horrible when 'tough times' keep happening over and over. Our heads may hurt and everybody and everything may seem unfair and rotten.

That's when the stress and *Knots* inside our bodies can grow bigger than our *Self-Control Power*. The alarm bell seems to grow 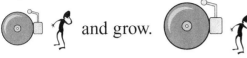 and grow and grow.

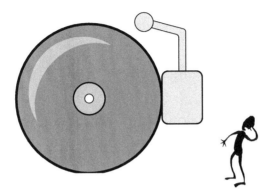

All of us, every man, woman, girl, and boy, have alarm systems inside of us. Our brains are made to keep us safe. So, when we sense danger, the inside of our brains starts sending 'danger' signals that act like alarm bells. For children and adults who have lived with scary or dangerous things happening, the alarm bells can be very loud and go on for a long time especially if they feel no one cares or they have no one who can help them. And, if the scary or dangerous things happen over and over, it may feel like no time is really safe and that the alarm bells will be ringing forever and ever and ever . . .

When the alarm bells are ringing loud, our brains go into survival mode to keep us alive. An inner part of our brains takes over to help us escape danger in four ways, sometimes called the '4 F's': Fight, Flee, Freeze, or Faint. We may hit or kick (Fight). We may run away (Flee). But if we can't fight and if we can't run away, we may run away in our minds (Freeze) and feel like we're not really there. Our bodies may be frozen, but in our minds, we may escape what seems too horrible to live through. And, when things are really, really bad, we may even fall down and pass out (Faint). Fleeing, Fighting, Freezing, or Fainting can help us survive in the short run, but, at the same time, we are so busy fighting, running away with our bodies, or running away in our minds that we can't use our whole brains. And, when this happens, we can't act as smart as we can really be. We also miss out on learning other ways to make things better.

That's also when it's easy to 'Blow your Top,' 'Lose your Mind,' and 'Get in Trouble,' even when you don't want to. It may feel like you can't turn the alarm off or stop thinking about the bad things that hurt you or people you care about. You may feel like the bad things are going to happen again and again, and that there is no one who will help you. Or, it may seem too hard to even say out loud what happened, so you can't even ask for help. And, the only thing you can do is to Hit, Kick, fight someone, , or if that doesn't work to Run Away, , or just Freeze and try to forget about everything and everybody.

That's when 'tough times' seem to take over our bodies, minds, and relationships. And, that is when 'tough times' can lead to traumatic stress.

SOS FOR STRESS

Heroes know that being hurt is part of real life. Bad things do happen. Sometimes good people get sick or get hurt or lose people they love. Heroes fight to make sure that the bad times don't take over what is good in our lives, so we don't have to live day after day with traumatic stress.

Heroes learn to use their minds and bodies to think and act, so they can make the world a little better for everyone. Even when 'tough times' seem horrible and impossible to change, heroes keep on trying. Heroes keep on working to find ways to make things better and stop traumatic stress from taking over our lives.

A hero knows that staying calm and in control is a skill that can be learned and improved step by step, day by day, year by year. It's very much like learning to ride a bike. It may seem hard or even impossible at first, but then, with a lot of practice, it becomes easier. You can grow your *Self-Control Power* and keep traumatic stress from taking over your mind and body by practicing skills using your breathing, your eyes, ears, and other senses, and your mind.

SOS for Stress[3] is one tool you can use to stay in control. *SOS for Stress* means taking three simple steps to reduce stress and make things better:

1. Slow down.
2. Open your eyes.
3. Seek help and help others.

The first step is to learn how to focus your mind and body so you can be in control to do what you want to do, to get where you want to go, and then to learn to do this anywhere you may be.

The second step is to open your eyes to who and what can help you. When bad things happen, it's easy to miss all the good things and good people that can help at home, at school, night or day, wherever you are.

SOS[4] for Stress

Slow down: Six-step breathing and body scan.

Open your eyes: Who and what can help?

Seek help and help others

Heroes use the tough times in their lives to learn, to grow, to help others, and to get help for themselves.

Kagan, R. (2017) *Real Life Heroes: Toolkit for Treating Traumatic Stress in Children and Families, 2nd Edition.* New York: Routledge.

The third step is to get help when you need it. Heroes know that no one succeeds very well alone. Heroes get help and give help. Heroes help other heroes.

Now comes the hard part. Saying it, even writing it down, isn't enough. You have to *do* it.

Just like learning to make a winning jump shot or play a guitar, it takes a lot of practice. And, sometimes, the more 'tough times' you've had, the more practice and help you need. It's like learning to ride a bike, or shoot a basket. At first, to a little child, it seems very hard. And, even a strong boy or girl may fail if they feel stressed. But then, with a lot of practice every day and a helpful guide, suddenly it clicks. You can do it. And, even better, you can do it when you *need* to do it to help you and the people you care about make things better.

So, let's practice *SOS for Stress*.[5]

SLOW DOWN

Slowly scan over your body from the tip of your toes through your feet, ankles, knees, thighs, hips, stomach, chest, arms, and up your neck to your mouth, and all over your head to the very top. It's OK whatever you are feeling. If you feel tight or tense anywhere, just notice it. Remember, your body is helping you by alerting you when you need to do something to make things better.

Now, see what happens when you focus your mind on your breathing. Breathe in and out, slower and slower. Count slowly (1, 2, 3) as you breathe in. Fill up your whole body from the tip of your toes to the top of your head, then let it go. Let the air flow back out as you count backwards slowly (3, 2, 1). It's like a circle. Breathe slowly in through your nose (1, 2, 3) and then let the air go back out slowly through your mouth (3, 2, 1).

It sometimes helps to imagine the air flowing in warm and gentle (as you count 1, 2, 3) until it touches any parts in your body that feel a little tight or tense. Then, when the air flows back out (3, 2, 1), it takes all the tightness away. You can also practice tightening your body as you breathe in (1, 2, 3) and then letting your body relax when you let the air out (3, 2, 1). Let each breath in bring air into your body to make you stronger and each breath out take away some of the knots in your body.

Practice doing this twice a day for a few minutes. It helps to have someone practice with you. The more you practice, the more control you develop to use your mind to do what you want to do. That's *Mind Power*.

If you find yourself thinking of something else, that's normal. Just bring your mind back and focus again on your breathing. It may help to think of your thoughts like water going down a river or like cars passing down your street. Thoughts keep on coming. That's normal. Just notice them and bring your mind gently back to your breathing. Every time you practice this, your mind power will grow stronger. And, you'll be better prepared to keep yourself calmer if things get tough.

OPEN YOUR EYES

Focus on 'right now,' in this place. Wiggle your toes. If you are sitting down, feel the chair holding you up. Notice who's around who could help you. Look for people you like and trust. Then, look for what's around you that could help; things that could help you stay calm and do what you need to do.

Sometimes, it may seem like you are all alone, that no one cares, or no one will help. Opening your eyes also means opening your mind and remembering people who helped you in the past. People who loved and cared about you.

Take a piece of paper and draw a picture of someone who made you feel warm, and good, and cared for. Or, draw a time when you remember feeling safe. After you draw this picture, close your eyes and see if you can bring it back into your mind. Try to picture it clearly. Try to remember how you felt in your body, how the people around you looked. Then, next time you practice your breathing, see if you can bring up this picture. See if you can bring that same feeling into your body as you breathe in (1, 2, 3).

SEEK HELP AND HELP OTHERS

Practice asking for help learning something. Ask someone in your family, a teacher, or a friend who knows how to do something you'd like to do better, such as making a jump shot, throwing a football, hitting a curve ball, figuring out how to use an app, learning to do algebra, or a magic trick. It can be something fun or something for school. Asking for help can make other people feel good. And, you can learn who is able and willing to help you. That way, if things get tough, you'll know who can help.

And, while you are trying this out, think about some ways you can help the people you care about. Do something that helps someone else. Help a younger child learn something you know how to do. Surprise someone. Then, notice how you feel when you help.

When 'tough times' happen, it's easy to forget all the *Self-Control Power* you have. To help you remember, make a *Power Card* that you can put in your pocket to take with you wherever you go.

Start by making a photocopy or cutting the card on the next page. In the top half of the card, draw someone who makes you feel safer and stronger or a special memory of a time when you felt safe. Paste your *SOS for Stress* card on a 3 × 5 index card to make it stronger, then fold the card in the middle and it's ready to go.[6] Whenever you feel stress (knots) in your body, pull out your card and remind yourself of this person or this safe time and how you can use SOS to feel better. If someone is helping you with this book, encourage them to make their own card.

Practice using *SOS for Stress* twice a day, every day, for a week. Just like athletes and musicians who practice sports or music skills every day, SOS practice will make your skills for self-control stronger. Practice using SOS in different places at least once a day. Try using SOS the next time you are about to take a test at school, play in a sports competition such as a basketball game, or when you muster the courage to dive off a high diving board, swim to the bottom of a deep pool, or ski down a double diamond ski slope. You can also use your SOS skills the next time there is a storm warning in your area. *SOS for Stress* can help you stay calmer everywhere you go, in *good times* and 'tough times'. It's all about using your mind *and* your body.

SOS[7] for Stress

Slow down: Six-step breathing and body scan.

Open your eyes: who and what can help?

Seek help and help others

Heroes use the tough times in their lives to learn, to grow, to help others, and to get help for themselves.

Kagan, R. (2017) *Real Life Heroes: Toolkit for Treating Traumatic Stress in Children and Families, 2nd Edition*. New York: Routledge.

Your senses can help you increase your self-control. Try these steps for each of your senses:[8]

Eyes:	Look at a photograph of someone or something that makes you feel peaceful. Look at plants or flowers. Find something in every room and every place you go that makes you feel good inside.
Ears:	Listen to relaxing music, or even the music in a favorite person's voice. Sing along with a 'feel-good' song. Tap a rhythm or play an instrument.
Taste buds:	Treat yourself to a tasty, soothing drink (e.g., hot chocolate or herbal tea, cold soda, ice cubes). Sip slowly, as slowly as you can, and discover how good it tastes.
Nose:	Sniff as you sip or pull out a favorite perfume or cologne that makes you feel good or remember someone you love. Sniff flowers, spices, or a favorite treat.
Touch:	Smooth a rich peaceful smelling lotion on your hand. Take a warm bubble bath, pet a friendly animal, rub a soft piece of fabric.

Your body is also designed to **move**. You can run, jump, dance, swim, or play sports. And, your body has a sense of **balance** and a sense of where you are that can help you when you move. Close your eyes and try leaning to the right, then to the left, without looking. Your brain can sense your position and tell you if you're lying down, standing up, tilted, or about to fall over. Go ahead, try it! And, if someone is helping you with this book, ask them to try it too. Like your other senses (smell, hearing, sight, touch, taste), your sense of balance can grow and help keep you balanced when you're standing, running, jumping, riding a bike, skating over ice, skiing fast down a bumpy hill.

Moving and balancing can help you feel calm. Draw a picture of something that you like to do to relax. If someone is helping you with this book, ask them to draw their own picture.

Later, try out some other ways you can use movement to help you feel better, even in 'tough times':

- ☐ Take a walk and focus on how you feel with each step.
- ☐ Swim, play a sport, or exercise.
- ☐ Learn and practice yoga or mindfulness.

Don't forget to get help from someone you trust:

- ☐ Talk to a friend.
- ☐ Hug someone you trust.

Write your favorite things to do to stay calm on the next page to make a safety plan. Make a photocopy of it and paste it on a 5 × 7 inch index card. Then, draw a picture on the other side of the card showing yourself using some of the ways you can stay calm and people who can help you feel safe and good. Put the card in your wallet, backpack, or pocket. If someone is helping you, encourage them to make their own card.

SAFETY FIRST

Three things I can do to stay calm

1. _____

2. _____

3. _____

My senses can help me:

Eyes: _____

Ears: _____

Taste buds: _____

Nose:_____

Touch: _____

Movement-balance:_____

People I can call for help (name and phone #):

_____

_____

_____

_____

_____

SAFETY FIRST CARD—FRONT

SAFETY FIRST CARD—BACK

Remember to keep practicing your breathing and your skills to calm down all five senses. Practice every day at home, at school, and wherever you go.

Each chapter of this workbook will give you more ways you can build your *Self-Control Power*, find people to help you, find people you can help, and reduce traumatic stress. Step by step, chapter by chapter, you can become stronger and stronger by working on the Heroes Challenge.

THE HEROES CHALLENGE

It's hard to face traumatic stress. In many ways, it may seem easier to stay feeling trapped or stuck, not daring to change. Heroes muster the courage to heal from their wounds and use what they learn to help other people who have to face 'tough times'.

Heroes use the 'tough times' in their lives to grow stronger.

Emotions and feelings are natural. Use them to grow smarter.

Relationships matter. Heroes work together to make things better.

Open up your options. Use the power of your brain to find new ways to solve problems with help from other people.

Experiment. Find the courage to check out and test out new solutions to old problems.

Stronger and **S**tronger. Discover your skills and make them even stronger. Remember who cared about you in the past and find people who care enough to help you grow.

Chapter 2

A Little About Me

This is a drawing or photograph of me doing something fun.

[If someone is helping you with this book, please encourage them to draw their own picture for this page and for all other pages in this book.]

These are some of the other things that I like to do for fun.

_____

_____

_____

_____

It is natural to have many feelings at different times. In the boxes below, draw how you show four feelings: happy, sad, fear, and anger.

These are drawings or photographs showing how I can feel kindness or caring, worried, calm, and brave.

Sometimes, we want other people to think we are feeling in a different way than we are really feeling. We may feel afraid on the inside but try to look cool and calm on the outside. Or, we may feel mad on the inside but pretend to look happy on the outside. Use colored markers or pencils to show different feelings and color in how you would like other people to think you were feeling right now.[1]

MY OUTSIDE FEELINGS[2]

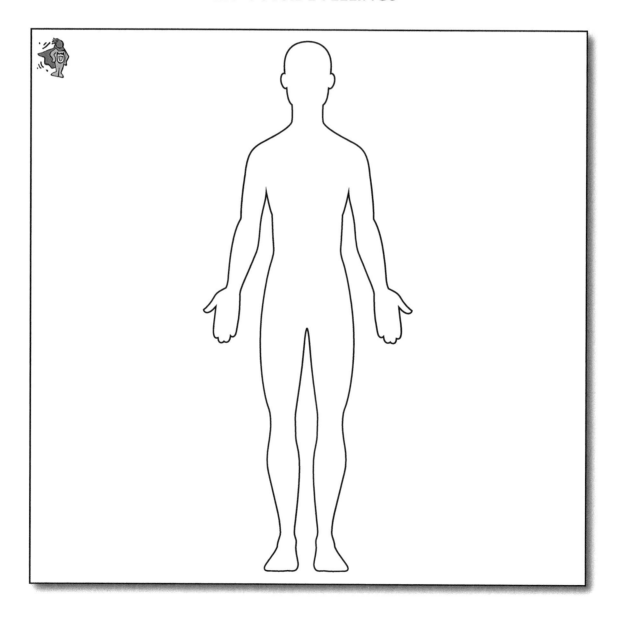

This is a drawing of how I'm *really* feeling on the inside right now.

[Pick a colored marker or pencil and color in how different parts of your body feel on the figure below.]

MY INSIDE FEELINGS

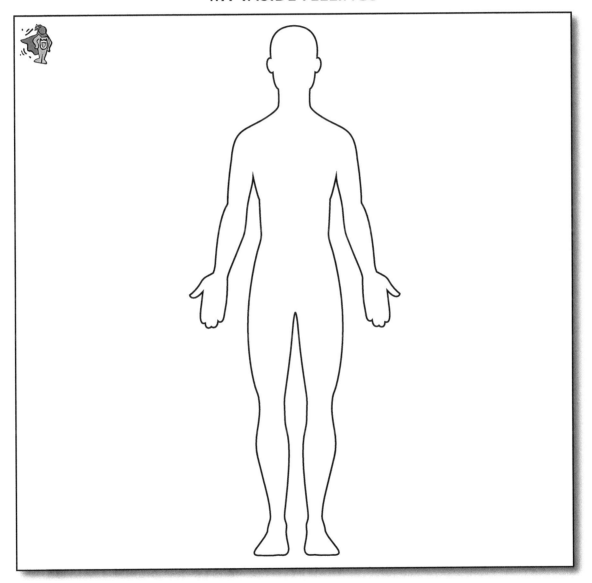

Chapter 3

Heroes

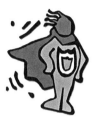 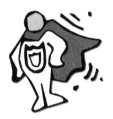

My favorite hero from a movie, TV show, or book is

_____

_____

I like how he/she helps people by

_____

_____

_____

_____

[Draw or cut out a picture of your hero doing something especially brave and put it below.]

My hero uses skills to help other people, including the ability to

_____

_____

Some people think that heroes are just fantasies.

But I know a real person who acted as a hero. This is what happened.

[Draw or write below a story of someone who helped someone or showed a special kind of courage.]

This person used skills to help others, including the ability to

_____

_____

These are some other people that I look up to because of the special things they do.

[List as many names as you like below or fill the page with photographs or drawings of something special each person does.]

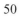

If my favorite hero from real life, movies, or books was with me now, this is what I would like to do.

_____

_____

_____

And then we would

_____

_____

_____

If I were driving in a car with my favorite hero, I would have a bumper sticker in the back showing how I would feel about myself. The bumper sticker would tell everybody

_____

_____

_____

My favorite hero and I would drive off and we would help people by

_____

_____

If I could make my own superhero Band-Aid, I would put in a picture of one of my favorite heroes. [Draw in your hero below.]

[Drawing box]

The great thing about this Band-Aid would be its power to heal any cut, wound, or pain. You could simply put the Band-Aid on a cut or wound, and then . . . [Write what would happen.]

_____

_____

_____

_____

_____

_____

If I was a hero in a movie, story, or book, this is what the movie poster would look like.

[Draw a picture or take a photograph of yourself acting in your movie.]

What special skills or powers would you have?

_____

_____

What would you be doing in the movie to help other people?

_____

_____

Every girl, boy, man, and woman needs help from time to time. That is just the way it is.

I remember helping other people when I was younger. I remember helping

_____

_____

I helped them by

_____

_____

Afterward, I thought to myself that I was

_____

_____

Helping made me feel

_____

_____

I remember one of the times in my life when I felt especially proud of what I did and how I helped someone. I was _____ years old. This is what I did.

_____

_____

_____

_____

_____

_____

_____

_____

Now that I am older, I know other ways to help people.

[Make a collage or draw pictures on the next page showing something you could do to make your home, your neighborhood, or your school better.]

Chapter 4

Power Plans

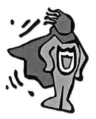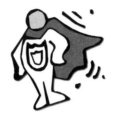

Think of how your favorite heroes use their skills and work together with others to cope with 'tough times'. Then, use the next pages to plan how you can make things better at home, at school, and in your town or city with help from people who care about you.[1]

REAL LIFE HEROES

Youth Power Plan

Name: _____   Age: _____   Date: _____

These are some special things about me (skills, talents, interests, things I like to do, what I'm proud of):

_____

_____

_____

There are some special people who are important to me, care for me, or help me learn important skills:

_____

_____

These are some of the best things that happened for me and my family:

Age   What Happened, Who Was with Me

_____   _____

_____   _____

_____   _____

_____   _____

_____   _____

_____   _____

These are some times I felt safe:

Age   What Happened, Who Was with Me

_____   _____

_____   _____

_____   _____

_____   _____

_____   _____

I think school is:

_____

School makes me feel:

_____

My favorite class or subject is:

_____

My worst class or subject is:

_____

It helps me learn when teachers:

_____

These are some things that have made me feel stressed or unsafe or remind me of bad times:

_____

_____

I also think some of these things[2] (below) get me feeling stressed:

☐ Feeling no one listens to me   ☐ Feeling pressured

☐ Being touched   ☐ Lack of privacy

☐ People yelling   ☐ Loud noises

☐ Feeling lonely   ☐ Arguments

☐ Not having control   ☐ Being alone

☐ Darkness   ☐ Being stared at

☐ Being teased   ☐ Feeling tired

☐ Feeling hungry   ☐ Being criticized

☐ Being reminded of a very   ☐ Being told 'no' about
   bad time in my life   something I want

☐ Particular people: _____

_____

☐ Particular time of day: _____

☐ Particular time of year: _____

☐ Other things that get me stressed [please describe]:

_____

_____

These are some things I do, show, or feel when I am starting to lose self-control [warning signs]:

_____

_____

I also find some of these things (below) happen when I am getting stressed:

☐ Stomach hurts   ☐ Breathing hard

☐ Racing heart   ☐ Clenching teeth

☐ Clenching fists   ☐ Sweating

☐ Wringing hands   ☐ Using loud voice

☐ Sleeping a lot   ☐ Trouble sleeping

☐ Acting hyper   ☐ Swearing

☐ Jittery legs   ☐ Rocking

☐ Can't sit still   ☐ Being rude

☐ Pacing   ☐ Crying

☐ Staring at something   ☐ Hurting things

☐ Eating more   ☐ Eating less

☐ Avoiding people or isolating   ☐ Laughing loudly

☐ Singing inappropriately

☐ Other [please describe]:

_____

_____

These are some of the things I have done when I was stressed that led to problems for me or other people:

_____

_____

_____

I have done some of these things (below) when I was stressed:

☐ Losing control   ☐ Leaving without permission

☐ Running away   ☐ Threatening others

☐ Hurting people   ☐ Hurting myself

☐ Attempting suicide   ☐ Using alcohol

☐ Using drugs   ☐ Getting into fights

☐ Other [please describe]:

_____

_____

These are some things that help me calm down and help me and other people feel safe in 'tough times':

_____

_____

_____

These are some of the other things that help me calm down:

☐ Talking with family members [who?]:

_____

☐ Talking with adults [who?]:

_____

☐ Talking with friends [who?]:

_____

☐ Time alone in my room   ☐ Listening to music

☐ Reading a book   ☐ Playing an instrument

☐ Walking   ☐ A quiet place

☐ Drawing/art   ☐ Molding clay

☐ Jokes/humor   ☐ Writing in a journal

☐ Hugging a stuffed animal   ☐ Exercising

☐ Cold washcloth on face   ☐ Drinking hot tea

☐ Drinking cold water   ☐ Deep breathing

☐ Taking a shower   ☐ Playing cards

☐ Video games   ☐ Lying down

☐ Meditating   ☐ Getting a hug

☐ Holding ice in hands   ☐ Using the gym

☐ Rocking chair   ☐ Praying

☐ Being around others   ☐ Being read a story

☐ Wrapping myself in something   ☐ Making a collage
   warm or soft

☐ Crying   ☐ Running

☐ Shooting baskets   ☐ Doing chores/jobs

☐ Yoga   ☐ Dancing

☐ Swimming

☐ Other [please specify]:

_____

_____

Draw a picture of how other people can help you calm down.

These are things that other people do that make me feel more stressed and do not help me calm down:

_____

_____

_____

Some of these things (below) also make me feel more stressed:

☐ Being left alone   ☐ Having to be with people

☐ Sarcasm   ☐ Being disrespected

☐ Not being listened to   ☐ Being ignored

☐ Loud tones of voice   ☐ Peers teasing

☐ Adults lecturing   ☐ Adults giving advice

☐ Being touched   ☐ Being reminded of the rules

☐ Other [please describe]:

_____

_____

My *Power Plan*

1. These are things I will do to keep myself calm, safe, and strong, all day and at night:

_____

_____

_____

_____

_____

This is how I will use my senses, my body, and my mind to help calm myself.[3] I will use:

(a) My eyes to _____

(b) My ears to _____

(c) My nose to _____

(d) My mouth to _____

(e) My hands and arms to _____

(f) My legs and feet to _____

(g) My mind to _____

2. I will watch for these warning signals in my body and my mind that tell me when I am getting stressed:

_____

_____

3. I would like caring adults to watch for warning signals I show by what I do, how my face looks, or how I talk, like when I:

_____

_____

4. These are people I can call for help, day or night [copy and cut out to take with you, or put into a smartphone if you have one]:

People I Trust	Names	Phone #s
Family members		
Other adults who take care of you		
Therapists, teachers, staff, county		
Friends		

5. When adults notice that I'm getting upset,[4] I would like them to help me feel better and stay safe by:

_____

_____

_____

6. I will help other people feel better and stay safe by:

_____

_____

_____

7. I will develop some of my special skills and talents by:

_____

_____

_____

8. I will practice this plan with help from:

_____

_____

_____

Youth signature: _____   Date: _____

Witnessed by: _____   Date: _____

                  _____   Date: _____

                  _____   Date: _____

Make a *Pocket Power Card* by filling in the lines below. For your goals, write in what is most important for you. Warning signs can be feelings in your body, like your stomach hurting or your foot swinging. Steps for Success are three things you can do to make things better. Then make a photocopy of the *Power Card*. Paste it on a 3 × 5 inch index card and draw a picture on the back (or attach a photo) that reminds you of a time when you felt safe with someone who cared about you. Take this card with you to remind you of the power you carry wherever you go.

REAL LIFE HEROES

Pocket Power Plan

My goals: _____

_____

My warning signs: _____

_____

Triple S (Step by Step to Success):

1. _____
2. _____
3. _____

With help from [name/phone #]:

1. _____
2. _____
3. _____

Adults can help me by:

_____

_____

POWER CARD—FRONT

POWER CARD—BACK

Chapter 5

My Family

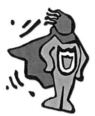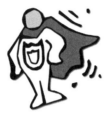

This chapter has questions about people who helped you when you were little. If you do not know the answers, that is perfectly OK. Sometimes it takes a detective to figure things out.

Who could help you find out? Who could you talk to, visit, or write a letter to? Who knows about you and the people who cared for you? [If you have trouble remembering people, it is a good idea to ask someone you trust, a parent, aunt, uncle, grandparent, or a counselor to help you find out. List below some people who you would talk to if you were a detective trying to learn about your life as a little boy/girl even before you were old enough to remember things.]

---

*   *   *

If I were a tree, my family and friends would be my roots, anchoring me to the soil and giving me water and nutrients.

[Write in the names of people in your family, special friends, any adoptive or foster parents or other adults who helped you, and any special pets. Then, darken in the lines (roots) leading from you to the most important people in your life.]

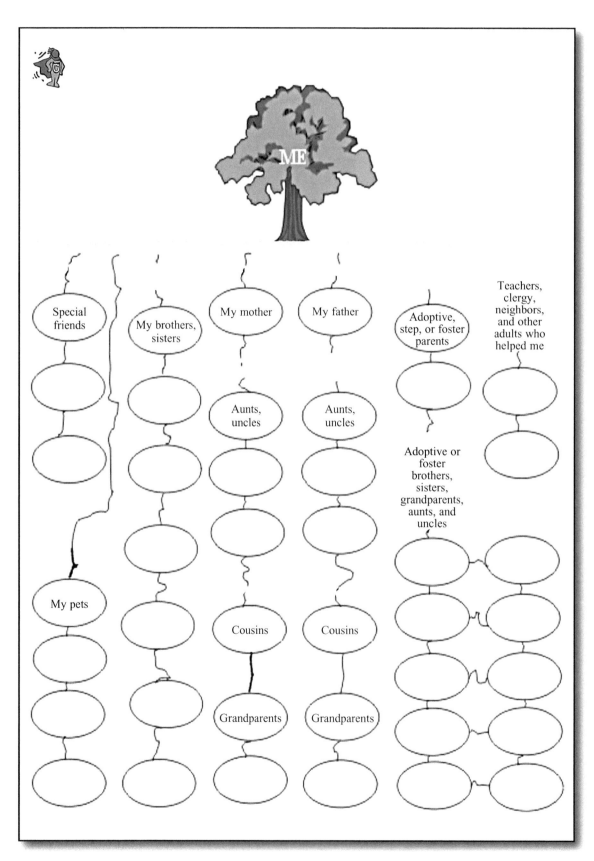

This is a picture of someone who took care of me before I was 2 years old.

[If you cannot remember who helped you, is there someone (an aunt, an uncle, a grandparent, an older sibling) you could ask?]

I found out that this person used to do some special things to help me, such as:

_____

_____

This is a person who took care of me when I was between 2 and 5 years old.

[Draw a picture the way you remember him or her.]

These are some of the special things he or she did for me:

_____

_____

This is a drawing or photograph of a person who helped me when I was older.

These are some of the special things he or she did for me:

_____

_____

These are some of the people I remember who helped me when I was sick.

[If you have trouble remembering, is there someone you could ask?]

_____

_____

_____

This is a picture of how they helped me.

This is a picture showing some of the people in my family who taught me ways to make things better.

[Draw these people or use photographs. Make a note next to each person, showing one thing he or she taught you that was helpful.]

When I was younger, I liked to visit

_____

_____

The best part of my visits was when I got to

_____

_____

When I grew older, I liked to visit

_____

_____

The best part of my visits was when I got to

_____

_____

These are some special people I would like to visit now.

_____

_____

This is what I would like to do with them.

_____

_____

This is a picture of something I like to do with my brothers, sisters, parents, aunts, uncles, cousins, or grandparents.

Here are some of the things these family members like the best about me.

_____

_____

If I really needed help, I would go to see

_____

_____

If I knocked on this person's door, he or she would say

_____

_____

And then, he or she would

_____

_____

[Draw a map below showing the roads you could take to get to this person, if you remember, or ask an adult to help you find out.]

Chapter 6

Important People

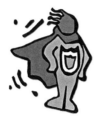 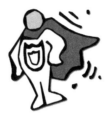

These are some of the things I like to do with friends.

_____

_____

_____

_____

If you asked my friends what they liked about me, they would
say I was

_____

_____

_____

_____

If my friends and I were in a movie or video game together, this is what would happen.

First,

_____

_____

_____

_____

_____

Then,

_____

_____

_____

_____

_____

_____

By the end of the movie, this is how we would make things better:

_____

_____

_____

_____

_____

_____

What I like to do best in school is

_____

_____

_____

_____

The hardest thing about school is

_____

_____

_____

_____

Here are the names of some of the people who helped me with schoolwork when I was younger:

_____

_____

_____

_____

Now, when I need it, these people help me with schoolwork:

_____

_____

_____

_____

These are some of the best times I remember in my whole life.

The best:

_____

I was _____ years old.

Second best:

_____

I was _____ years old.

Third best:

_____

I was _____ years old.

Fourth best:

_____

I was _____ years old.

Fifth best:

_____

I was _____ years old.

The people who helped make these times so good were

_____

_____

_____

My most special holiday (or birthday) was when

_____

_____

I celebrated with

_____

_____

The best part of our celebration was when

_____

_____

If I had the power to declare a new holiday,[1] my own special celebration day, I would call it

_____

_____

And I would like to have these people join me to celebrate:

_____

_____

The best part of this celebration would be

_____

_____

[Draw how you would celebrate below or imagine yourself dancing and show how you would move about the page with swirls and colors. Then, write the name of your celebration at the top.]

MY CELEBRATION

If I was running for president, this is what my campaign button would say.

[Draw in a button below with your name on it.]

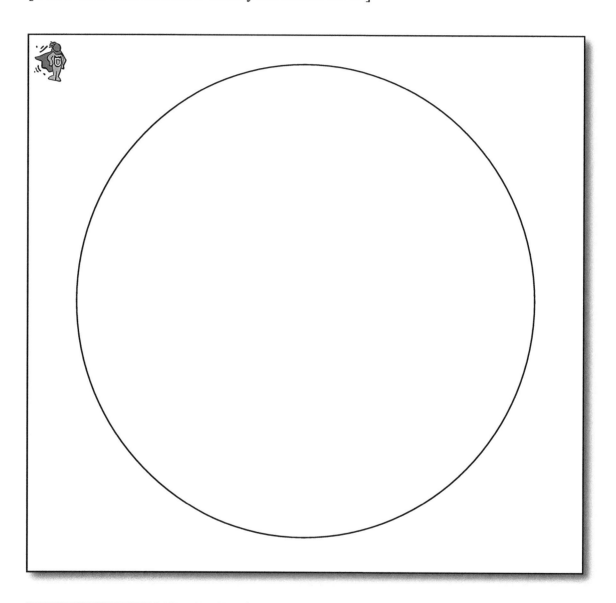

My campaign bumper sticker would tell everyone some of the good things I would do to make things better, such as how I

_____

_____

Chapter 7

Mind Power

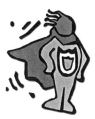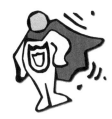

Some people think that it takes magic to make things better when things get tough and that only a wizard can do magic.

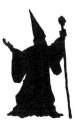

But, real magicians know that behind every magic trick is a secret, the trick that makes the magic work. Magicians practice the tricks behind the magic over and over to make it look as easy as saying "abracadabra."

What magic tricks do you know? What can you do?

_____

_____

_____

_____

How did you learn your magic tricks?

_____

_____

_____

_____

If you had all the powers of the universe, what would you do to make things better for yourself and the people you care most about?

_____

_____

_____

_____

_____

MIND POWER

Mind Power means being able to keep yourself calm enough to figure out ways to make things better with help from other people. Like a magic trick, *Mind Power* means developing skills and it takes practice to make these skills work. It means knowing that feelings and thoughts come and go like waves in the ocean or leaves floating down a stream. It means finding ways to help you train your brain to get better at concentrating and solving problems. That doesn't mean you won't get distracted or upset sometimes. Everyone does. *Mind Power* helps you bring your attention back to what you want to focus on like a telescope[1] focuses on a distant planet. The more you practice bringing your mind back to focus,[2] the stronger your *Mind Power* gets. *Mind Power* helps you to calm yourself enough to adjust the controls of your telescope so you can see what is going on, to think about what is happening, to get help from other people when you need it, to come up with new plans to make things better, and to keep going if things get tough.

In this chapter, you can develop skills to calm your mind and body enough, so that you can help make things better in your life and the lives of the people you care about.

This is a picture of a time and a place where I felt safe and peaceful.

[If this is hard to remember, just think of a place where you felt even a little bit more relaxed and safe.]

I was [Where were you? Was anyone with you?]

_____

_____

_____

_____

What made it so peaceful was that

_____

_____

_____

_____

[Practice bringing this picture into your mind several times a day. When your mind starts to float away, bring your attention back to your picture. Think of your mind working like a powerful telescope helping you see the colors, sense the smells, hear the sounds and hold the feelings that go with your picture. You can aim your telescope where you want. Practice bringing up your picture of this time when you felt safe and peaceful along with using 'SOS' or your Power Plan when you start to feel just a little bit stressed. Keep practicing bringing up your picture until you can bring it up in your mind even when you are very stressed.]

This a picture of someone who helped me feel warm and good inside.

[It could be someone you remember from long ago or someone you know now].

What makes this memory so powerful is that

_____

_____

_____

_____

[Practice bringing this picture into your mind several times a day like you did with picture of your 'Safe Place.' When your mind starts to float away, bring your attention back. Imagine your mind working again like a powerful telescope helping you see the colors, sense the smells, hear the sounds and hold the feelings that go with your picture.]

When I am a little upset, this is what I do to help myself feel calm and safe.

_____

_____

Sometimes, my friends or family help me feel better. This is what they do.

_____

_____

When I am very upset, this is what I do to help me feel better. [Draw a picture below.]

What helps me the most is:

_____

_____

Sometimes, heroes think they have to be perfect, but the truth is that every girl, boy, man, and woman makes mistakes, lots of them. Real heroes make mistakes. Some mistakes are accidents, things that happen that were not planned. Sometimes, our mistakes were things we meant to do that turned out badly. And, sometimes, our mistakes hurt other people. When this happens, heroes may feel badly and try to hide their mistakes so no one will know. But, hiding mistakes can make us feel alone, nervous about being 'found out,' and even more embarrassed or ashamed about what we did. Hiding mistakes can make things much worse.

Heroes learn there is another way. They learn the difference between hurting someone else by accident or 'on purpose.' Accidents can often happen when people have lots of stress (Knots), without anyone planning to do something that hurts someone. Doing something 'on purpose' means thinking and planning what to do and then doing it.

Heroes learn that they can share what they did wrong with people they can trust. That takes courage. And, the great thing about sharing their mistakes is that it makes them stronger. They don't have to hide what they did. They don't have to worry about what they have done or blame themselves for being bad. And then, it is easier to get help from people they trust and find ways to make things better.

If the mistake was an accident, heroes can try to help the person who was hurt and lower their stress (Knots) so the mistake does not happen again. If the mistake was something that was done 'on purpose,' heroes can still try to make up as much as they can for what happened. They can fix or replace things that were broken. They can do nice things to help anyone who was hurt by what they did. They can also change what they do in the future so the mistake doesn't happen again.

That's the difference between pretend heroes and real heroes. Real heroes make mistakes and then use their courage to admit what they did, to share how sorry they feel, and to find a way to make things better with the help of other people.

Mistakes are not all bad. We can learn from our mistakes. Our mistakes also let us find out who will love us, even if we are not perfect. Our mistakes also remind us not to expect other people to be perfect because no one is.

Think of a hero you admire. What was one of the mistakes he or she made that hurt someone else?

_____

_____

Was the mistake an accident or 'on purpose'?

_____

_____

How did they feel after they made the mistake?

_____

_____

What did they do to make things better?

_____

_____

What was one mistake you made that hurt someone accidentally?

_____

_____

[Draw a picture below of how you tried to make things better after you made that mistake.]

In olden days, knights carried shields to protect them. They put pictures on those shields to remind them of how their skills, their families, and their heritage gave them strength when they were afraid. Draw on the shield below what helps you feel brave enough to share your mistakes with people you trust and keep trying to make things better, even when you feel afraid.

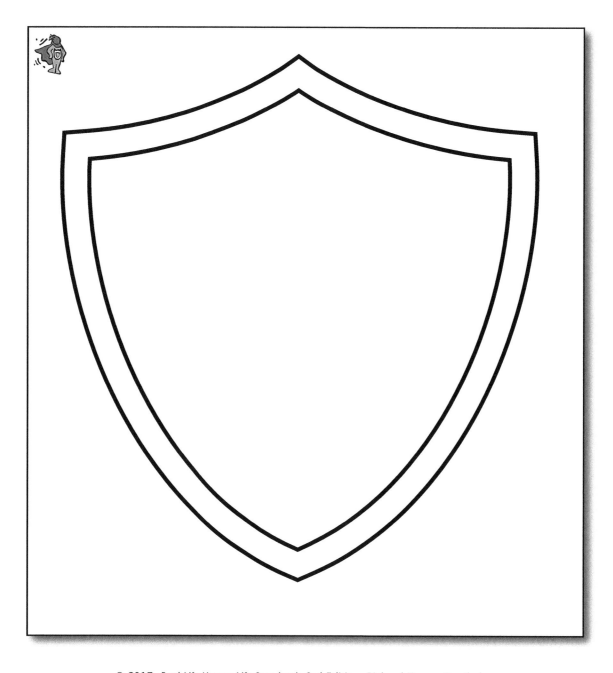

HOW I FEEL[3]

[Show on the thermometers below how you feel right now as you work on your Life Storybook. '0' would mean nothing at all. '10' would mean as much as you could ever feel of that feeling and '5' would be in the middle. So on the *Knots* thermometer, '0' would mean feeling calm and peaceful and '10' would mean feeling as upset (stressed) and terrible as you could ever feel. On the *Self-Control Power* thermometer, '0' would mean feeling unable do what you need to do to stay safe and do what you want to do, and '10' would mean feeling you could do what you need to do and stay safe.]

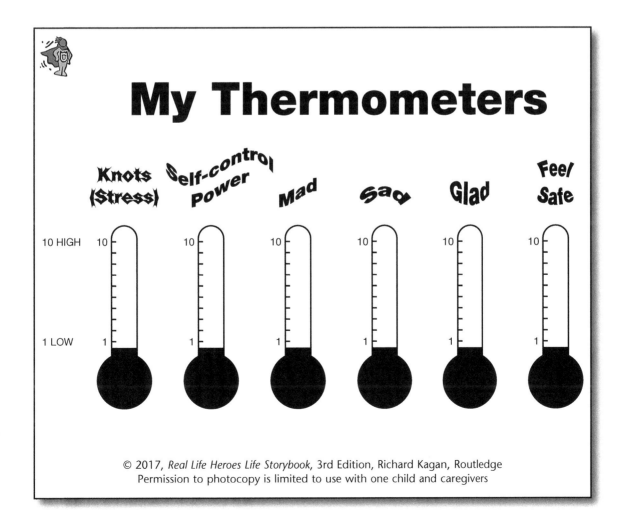

Chapter 8

Changing the Story

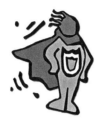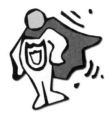

'Tough times' can make girls and boys, men and women, feel like nothing helps, that everything bad is their fault, that they are all alone, or, that nothing can change. And, thinking this way can make things even worse.

Here's how an "A" for "Alarm" can turn into an "F" for "Failing," faster than you can say A, B, C.

A*larm*: Sometimes bad things happen that make us feel all knotted up and stressed inside, like a close friend getting hurt badly in a football game after you tackled him, or if you heard your mom and dad screaming at each other, getting into another fight, the front door slamming and someone leaving, or if you heard someone you love is in the hospital and may die. And, the Knots can keep growing. Maybe your mom or dad complains that your room is a mess again and you didn't do what they asked. And, worse, they look so mad like you did something terrible. It may feel like your school's emergency alarm bell is going off inside your body. Only you may be the only one who hears it. Then, at school that day, a teacher looks angry and blames you for something you didn't do in front of the whole class.

Body Reaction: Your brain's self-defense system kicks in. It's battle time. Your heart is pounding. Your fists clench. Your stomach is one giant knot. The alarm bell has grown louder and louder and you can't turn it off. Before you know it, you slam your fist on your desk and start yelling at your teacher.

Catastrophic thinking: Your brain starts spinning: "That teacher hates me." "School stinks!" "Everybody is unfair to me."

Distress: Your body feels all tensed up, like a rope full of knots. Fears and anger shut down your power to think, to figure things out. Another part of your brain signals that it's time to fight, to run away, or to just go away somewhere in your mind and forget everything around you.

Emptiness: Afterward, it's like: "Nobody cares." "I'm all alone." "They all hate me." "They think I'm no good." "Maybe I am really 'no good.'" Your stomach may ache. Your head may feel like it is spinning. You may feel you don't have much air in your chest. Your body starts slumping down . . .

Failing: Everyone seems to be looking at you. Your mom or dad says you didn't do what they asked and something bad happened. Or, your teacher tells you to go to the principal's office. You know what that means, more time in the 'in-school suspension' room, or even suspension from school, and a note to bring home about "Fighting", "Disrupting the class," or "Failing to listen to teachers."

A TO F

When the *ABC's of Trauma* happen over and over and over, the "F" for "Failing" starts to feel like a way of life. It may feel like you are stuck in a bad movie that always ends the same rotten way. It's easy to start believing that:

"Everybody hates me."

"I can't win."

"I must be bad . . . no good . . . crazy . . . unlovable . . . and everybody knows it!"

It's as if the director of your movie yells "ACTION," but the same old story happens over and over. Every beginning starts to feel and look like an "A" for "Alarm" that leads to an "F" for Failing. Every day feels like a failing day. Every feeling seems too much, too bad, and too much to handle.

And, when 'tough times' keep happening over and over, it's easy to feel stuck. It may feel like you've fallen into a deep muddy pit and it's beginning to rain. And, every time you feel yourself falling into the pit, the pit feels deeper and deeper. The worse you feel, the more you try to fight, or run away, or just go off somewhere in your mind, but nothing seems to work. Feeling knotted up and out of control makes it harder and harder to climb out of the pit.

That's when you can start feeling like there is no escape, like you are stuck in a bad movie, and that nothing can help. It may feel like you are *Trapped in a Trauma Pit*. The bad feelings load you down, like rocks on top of your head and inside your body. You may feel like you are tied up in Knots that go up and down your body from your toes to your fingertips. Your stomach starts to burn and your head may get so tight it feels like it's being squeezed in a vise and about to explode.

MAKING THINGS BETTER

To get out of the *Trauma Pit*, heroes know that you need to use all your mind and body power, get help from other people, and grow stronger than all the bad feelings that keep knocking you down into that deep muddy pit.

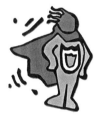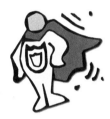

To find a way out, it helps to know how you got in. It's just like a magic trick. When you know how the trick works, you own the power of the magic.

And, when bad things keep happening, you can use *Mind Power*, the power of your brain, to make things better. Try this out and see if you can change the *ABC's of Trauma* with a couple tricks.

A_larm_: What was one 'tough time' that happened to you, something that made you feel just a little bad, no more than a '2' or '3' on the _Knots_ (_Stress_) scale or just a little more stressed than you usually feel? _____

_____

B_ody reactions_: What was your first reaction? How did you feel the alarm bells going off in your body?

_____

_____

What are some of the first clues inside your body when you have been reminded of 'tough times'?

_____

_____

C_atastrophic thinking_: When 'tough times' happened, what did you think this meant about you?

"I thought I was:

_____

_____ "

"Other people thought I was:

_____

_____ "

D_istress_: How did your thoughts and beliefs make you feel inside?

_____

_____

How high were you on the *Knots* scale (0–10)? _____

How much *Self-Control Power* (0–10) did you have? _____

Emptiness: Did anyone know how you felt?

_____

_____

Did anyone help?

_____

_____

Who could have helped, even just a little bit?

_____

_____

Failing: Did you stay in control?

_____

Were you able to achieve what was most important for you?

_____

_____

You can use your answers to these questions to figure out a better way to handle the "A" for "Alarm" and all the feelings that come with it. And, just like figuring out the secrets of a magic trick, figuring out the ABC's takes away the power of 'tough times' and helps make you stronger than your fears.

FEELING UP, FEELING DOWN, FEELINGS ALL AROUND

Mind Power helps us think about how feelings help us and use our feelings to make things better.

Heroes know that life means special days and not so special, or even not so good days, good times, and not so good times. It takes courage to accept that sometimes, bad things do happen, even to good people. In fact, bad things happen to everybody sooner or later.

Feelings are not 'bad' or 'good,' they are *just* feelings. And, feelings change. We may feel happy and then scared, mad and then sad.

Sometimes feelings show us the way our bodies learned to react to things that happened a long time ago, maybe even a time when we were so young that we can't remember what happened. Our feelings can give us clues to what upset us when we were younger and what is upsetting us now. And, knowing what upset us can help us figure out what can help make things better.

The first step is learning to be aware of our feelings. Some people think of feelings and worries like waves[1] rolling on to a beach. It may help to imagine yourself sitting on a bluff overlooking the ocean, higher than any wave could ever reach. Waves may look big at first and crash on to the shore; but soon, even the biggest waves fade out to sea. Waves come and go, just like our feelings. We can notice them and know that very soon another feeling will come, just like another wave flowing on to the sandy beach and again fading away while we sit high above, safely noticing each feeling or thought come and go.

Our alarm bells are part of our brains that are meant to help us in 'tough times'. Alarm bells signal that it's time for some action. Just like a movie director calling out "Action" at the start of a scene. The alarm bells may lead us to feel knotted up, scared, mad, or sad.

Heroes know *that feelings come and feelings go*, but *what you think and what you do is up to you*.

You can make things better by changing what happens after the "A" for "Alarm."

CHANGING THE STORY

You can become the director of your own story, just like the director of a movie. To change the story, heroes use the *Power of Their Brains for Thinking, Awareness, and Self-Control*. This is *Mind Power*, you can change what you pay attention to, how you think about what happened, and how you use the skills and strengths you have. With *Mind Power*, you can change how the story (or movie) goes.

Every movie has a script that tells the actors how to think, what feelings to show, and what to say. You can find the script of your story by taking another look at the ABCs:

Action: Drawing what happened, putting it to music, acting it out with some movement, and writing it down makes you the director. Drawings, music, and movement change how we pay attention to something and change what we see, hear, and feel. Drawings, music, and movement can give us clues to figure out how to solve a problem.

Try this out by drawing below a picture of that same 'tough time' when your *Knots* went up to a '2' or '3.'

What happened before your inner alarm went off?

_____

_____

Bodily reaction: Draw your true feelings below[2] with different colors for each feeling.

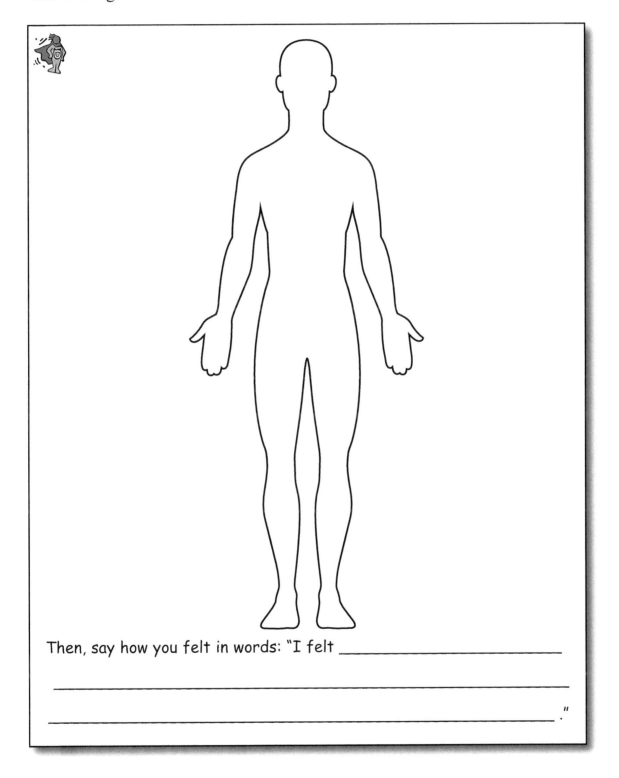

Then, say how you felt in words: "I felt _____

_____

_____. "

In your new story, you can change the "C" for "Catastrophic Thinking" to "C" for "Courage." But, first, you'll need to have all the powers of your brain working for you. This is where SOS[3] for Stress (from Chapter 1) and your Pocket Power Plan (from Chapter 2) can help.

Slow down

Open your eyes

Seek help and help others

Slowing down means learning how to focus your mind and body so you can be in control to do what you want to do, even when the alarm bells are going off. Mindfulness and yoga exercises can help you grow the power of your mind to stay focused on what you need to do to make things better. With every wave of stress, you can use *Mind Power* to bring your mind gently back to focus on things that calm yourself down. Think of your mind like a telescope. You can focus on any star or any thought, feeling, or part of your body.

Focusing on your breathing in, counting slowly (1, 2, 3) and then letting our breath out (3, 2, 1) can help. The more you practice bringing your mind back to your breathing, the stronger your *Mind Power* will become. Using your SOS Picture Power Card and Pocket Power Plan Card can also help.

Try this out as you practice your SOS:

Focus your attention on breathing in and out.

Let your thoughts or fears roll in like the waves[4] at a beach. Think of yourself high up on a bluff watching the waves flow in. Remember that every thought or feeling, like every wave, will fade away, no matter how big or scary it seems. Just notice the feeling or the thought as you breathe in counting slowly (1, 2, 3) and then let it go as you breathe out counting (3, 2, 1).

Practice breathing in ways that help you relax and feel good. Place one arm over your stomach and one arm over your chest as you breathe.[5] Try smiling just a little as you breathe. And, picture in your mind a time you felt safe and warm and cared for, like the picture you drew in Chapter 7 for a Safe Place or the picture on your *Pocket Power Card*.

Courageous thinking: Once our bodies are slowed down, we can turn on the power of our thinking.

Did what happen before your alarm bells went off involve people who looked, sounded, or acted like people who were going to hurt you or someone you loved?

_____

_____

Who were you reminded of?

_____

_____

Did what happen before your alarm bells went off involve places or things that reminded you of a 'tough time' where you were scared or hurt, or where someone you loved was scared or hurt?

_____

_____

What places or things or times in your life were you reminded of?

_____

_____

What would you like to happen to make things better for the situation you described when your alarm bells went off?

_____

_____

Now that your are older, smarter, and stronger, what could you or other people do to help make things better?

_____

_____

If that happened, what would you think about yourself?

"I could _____

_____ "

Test out your thinking by taking a look at what you wrote (page 111) about "Catastrophic Thinking" and how "I was . . ."

Was this really true? _____

Does believing this help or get in the way? _____

What would you rather believe about yourself?

"I am _____."

"I am good at: (1) _____; (2) _____."

"I like how I can: (1) _____; (2) _____."

Check off each of the following beliefs that you would like to be true for you:

☐ "I have been through 'tough times' before and I can get through them again if I have to."

☐ "I can help other people."

☐ "Deep down, I really do care about other people."

☐ "I have people who care about me."

☐ "Deep down, I know that I am a good person."

Now, go back and put a double check mark for each of those beliefs that are already true for you.

In your story, you can change the "D" from "Distress" to a "D" for "Defeating Traumatic Stress." You can't change what happened in the past, but you can change what you pay attention to, what you think, and what you do.

Defeating traumatic stress: Some children remind themselves of people who love them by pulling out photographs or special gifts such as a ring or a special stone. Some people relax by playing an instrument, talking to a friend, or taking slow breaths. Other children listen to a special song, walk in a special place, or remember a very special time when they felt safe and loved and peaceful.

What makes you feel better?

"I like to _____

_____."

What can help you relax and lower your *Knots*?

_____

_____

What helps you build your *Self-Control Power*?

_____

_____

SOS for Stress also means opening your eyes to who and what can help you. Heroes get help and give help.

With help from other people you trust, you can change the "E" for "Emptiness" and end your story with an "E" for "Excellence" instead of an "F" for "Failing."

Excellence

Who cared about you when you were little?

_____

Who cares about you now?

_____

Who will listen to you when you need to talk to someone?

_____

Who can give you good advice to make things better?

_____

Heroes seek help and help others. Who can you help?

_____

What could you do to help those people?

_____

Now, put together everything you've learned to change the ending of the story you started on page 106 with the alarm you felt. Draw on the next page how you could make things better using your *Mind Power* and getting help from people you can trust.

Knowing how the ABC's work helps you build your skills and find solutions. However, saying something, even writing it down, isn't enough. You have to do it.

Some skills may seem hard to learn. And, just like learning to make a winning jump shot or play a guitar, it takes practice. Athletes and musicians practice for hours every day. *Mind Power* takes a lot of practice. It helps to practice *Mind Power* and *SOS for Stress* every day. The more you practice, the better you get.

It's like learning to ride a bike. At first, to a little child, it seems impossible, but then, with a lot of practice and a helpful guide, it suddenly clicks. That's when the magic happens.

You can learn to use *Mind Power* and *SOS for Stress* wherever you go. You can use them in good times and 'tough times', just like you learned to ride a bike and keep your balance on sunny days or when it's raining. And, using these skills can help you change what happens in your life, the story of your life.

HEROES STORIES

Every hero story begins with someone who has been hurt, a boy or a girl, a man or a woman. Wounds can make us stronger or weaker and leave us with scars that remind us of what happened. It is good to know that scar tissue is tough. But unhealed wounds mean that the infection is still there.

Heroes muster the courage to heal from their wounds. They learn to use the power of their minds and the feelings in their bodies. And, heroes use what they learn to help others who face the same 'tough times'.

Remember the Heroes Challenge from Chapter 1:

Healing means using the pain in our lives to grow stronger instead of running away, lashing out at others, or hurting ourselves.

Emotions are natural. Celebrate them, use them to develop strengths and alert you that something needs to be done. To find your true feelings, take time to slow down, listen to your body, and check what is real.

Relationships matter. Heroes work together to make things better. Who would you want to help you? Real life heroes get help from other people (friends, family members, teachers, mentors).

Open up your options. Use the power of your brain to find new ways to solve problems. Check out your beliefs and change from catastrophic to courageous thinking. How would other heroes solve your problem?

Experiment: Muster the courage to check out and test out new solutions to problems. Courage can be learned but it takes practice. Skills take practice, but we can all learn. Mistakes mean we're learning. Heroes get knocked down and then get back up and try again.

Stronger and **S**tronger: Find your skills and increase them. Remember who cared about you in the past and find people who care enough to help you grow—people who won't knock you down. Move from strength to strength to help yourself and other people.

If you are ready for the next step in the Heroes Challenge, it's time to go to Chapter 9.

Chapter 9

Looking Back

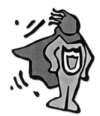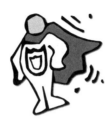

Our lives can look like roadmaps showing the places we have lived. Some of us have lived in one family and one home all our lives. And, some of us have moved so many times that our roadmaps can look like a maze. It may be hard to remember what really happened at different times in our lives. It helps to have a map and a list of places we've lived so we can see how our life stories fit together.

I was born in _____ [city/state]

I was born on _____ [month/day/year]

Now, I live in _____ [city/state]

Today's date is _____ [month/day/year]

That makes me _____ years old.

On the next page, draw a circle for every place you have lived, starting with where you were born. Write in the addresses if you remember them. Then connect each place with roads leading from home to home, all the way to where you live now.

Don't worry about how long each road is or whether you can remember the names of every home or place. Make your map as neat or as messy as you want. You could also cut out a map or print a map from a computer and highlight where you have lived and the roads connecting each home.

MY ROADMAP

Some of us have moved from home to home, and sometimes in and out of families or other places where children live. It is good to keep a record[1] so we do not get mixed up. This is detective work, discovering what happened from the day we were born until now.

You may have to ask adults you trust to help you figure out all the places you have lived and to help you find out what really happened. Use as many of the next pages as you need and leave spaces blank to fill in later as you learn more about the places you've lived. You can also copy a blank page and add extra pages if you lived in more than 10 places.

When I was _____ [years old], I lived in _____ [name of the city or town] with _____ _____ [the people who took care of me].

I often felt great/pretty good/bad/terrible [circle one of these feelings] living in this home.

I remember being told that the reason I needed to move was because

_____

_____

Now that I am older, I think that the reason I had to move was because

_____

_____

[Draw a picture or paste a photo of you or you and the people you lived with at this place below.]

When I was _____ [years old], I lived in _____
[name of the city or town] with _____
_____ [the people who took care of me].

I often felt great/pretty good/bad/terrible [circle one of these
feelings] living in this home.

I remember being told that the reason I needed to move was because

_____

_____

Now that I am older, I think that the reason I had to move was
because

_____

_____

[Draw a picture or paste a photo of you or you and the people you lived
with at this place below.]

When I was _____ [years old], I lived in _____ [name of the city or town] with _____ _____ [the people who took care of me].

I often felt great/pretty good/bad/terrible [circle one of these feelings] living in this home.

I remember being told that the reason I needed to move was because

_____

_____

Now that I am older, I think that the reason I had to move was because

_____

_____

[Draw a picture or paste a photo of you or you and the people you lived with at this place below.]

When I was _____ [years old], I lived in _____
[name of the city or town] with _____
_____ [the people who took care of me].

I often felt great/pretty good/bad/terrible [circle one of these feelings] living in this home.

I remember being told that the reason I needed to move was because

_____

_____

Now that I am older, I think that the reason I had to move was because

_____

_____

[Draw a picture or paste a photo of you or you and the people you lived with at this place below.]

When I was _____ [years old], I lived in _____
[name of the city or town] with _____
_____ [the people who took care of me].

I often felt great/pretty good/bad/terrible [circle one of these
feelings] living in this home.

I remember being told that the reason I needed to move was because

_____

_____

Now that I am older, I think that the reason I had to move was
because

_____

_____

[Draw a picture or paste a photo of you or you and the people you lived
with at this place below.]

When I was _____ [years old], I lived in _____
[name of the city or town] with _____
_____ [the people who took care of me].

I often felt great/pretty good/bad/terrible [circle one of these feelings] living in this home.

I remember being told that the reason I needed to move was because

_____

_____

Now that I am older, I think that the reason I had to move was because

_____

_____

[Draw a picture or paste a photo of you or you and the people you lived with at this place below.]

When I was _____ [years old], I lived in _____
[name of the city or town] with _____
_____ [the people who took care of me].

I often felt great/pretty good/bad/terrible [circle one of these
feelings] living in this home.

I remember being told that the reason I needed to move was because

_____

_____

Now that I am older, I think that the reason I had to move was
because

_____

_____

[Draw a picture or paste a photo of you or you and the people you lived
with at this place below.]

When I was _____ [years old], I lived in _____
[name of the city or town] with _____
_____ [the people who took care of me].

I often felt great/pretty good/bad/terrible [circle one of these
feelings] living in this home.

I remember being told that the reason I needed to move was because

_____

_____

Now that I am older, I think that the reason I had to move was
because

_____

_____

[Draw a picture or paste a photo of you or you and the people you lived
with at this place below.]

When I was _____ [years old], I lived in _____
[name of the city or town] with _____
_____ [the people who took care of me].

I often felt great/pretty good/bad/terrible [circle one of these
feelings] living in this home.

I remember being told that the reason I needed to move was because

_____

_____

Now that I am older, I think that the reason I had to move was
because

_____

_____

[Draw a picture or paste a photo of you or you and the people you lived
with at this place below.]

When I was _____ [years old], I lived in _____
[name of the city or town] with _____
_____ [the people who took care of me].

I often felt great/pretty good/bad/terrible [circle one of these feelings] living in this home.

I remember being told that the reason I needed to move was because

_____

_____

Now that I am older, I think that the reason I had to move was because

_____

_____

[Draw a picture or paste a photo of you or you and the people you lived with at this place below.]

These are some of the most important things that happened in my life. [Please circle how good or bad things were for you each year on a scale from 0 to 4, with 0 meaning 'the worst' and 4 'the best.']

Age	Important Things That Happened to Me or My Family	My Life Was a
0-1		0 1 2 3 4
1		0 1 2 3 4
2		0 1 2 3 4
3		0 1 2 3 4
4		0 1 2 3 4
5		0 1 2 3 4
6		0 1 2 3 4
7		0 1 2 3 4
8		0 1 2 3 4
9		0 1 2 3 4
10		0 1 2 3 4
11		0 1 2 3 4
12		0 1 2 3 4
13		0 1 2 3 4
14		0 1 2 3 4
15		0 1 2 3 4
16		0 1 2 3 4
17		0 1 2 3 4
18		0 1 2 3 4

Chapter 10

Through the 'Tough Times'[1]

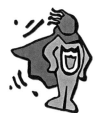 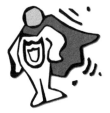

Every boy, girl, man, and woman has 'tough times' in their lives. This is a story of how I got through the first 'tough time' in my life. I am going to draw this story with five pictures that, together, make a story that begins before the 'tough time' and ends at a time when the 'tough time' was over and I felt safer and better. This story has five chapters, one for every picture, and if you put them all together, it works like a movie that goes from picture to picture and ends with the safer and better time.

[Start by drawing Chapter 2 of your story, the second box, which shows what happened in the 'tough time'. You can add words and feelings later. For now, keep going and draw Chapters 3 and 4. Then, go back and draw Chapter 1, which shows what happened *before* the 'tough time'. To finish your story, draw Chapter 5, which shows some of the things you learned from getting through your tough time and how you and the people who care about you can make things better now that your are older, smarter, and stronger. If this seems confusing or you don't remember what happened, ask someone you trust to help you do these stories. And remember, for every story, you will *always* end up at the part where things are safer and better.]

[Remember to start on the next page with Chapter 2 of your story.
After you draw pictures for Chapters 2, 3, and 4, then draw below what
happened *before* the 'tough time'.]

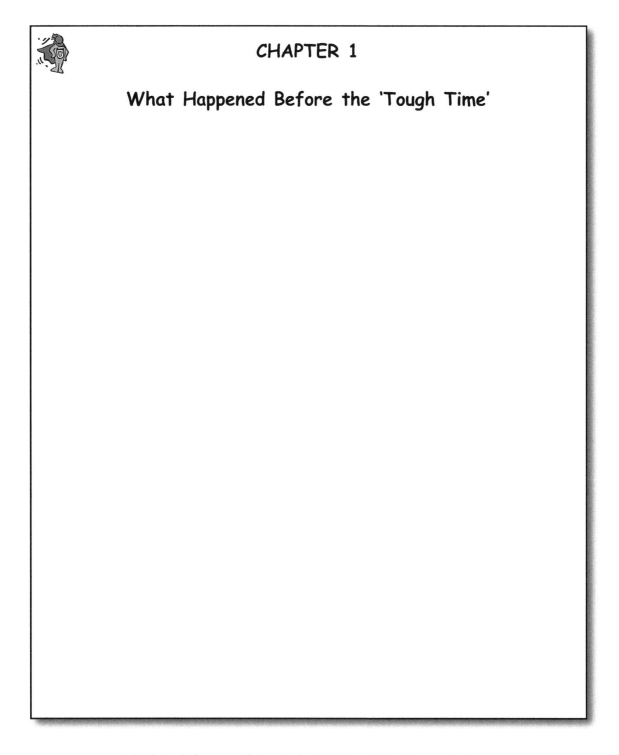

[Draw what happened in the box below.]

CHAPTER 2

The 'Tough Time'

[Next, show what you and other people did that helped you get through the 'tough time'.]

CHAPTER 3

What Helped Make Things Better

[Next, draw a time when things were better, when you felt safer and the 'tough time' was over. This can be right after the 'tough time', or months or years later.]

CHAPTER 4

A Better Time

[Go back four pages to draw Chapter 1 of your story, then come back to this page and think about how you are now older, stronger, and smarter. Draw below what you and people who care about you could do to make things better if the 'tough time' started to happen again.]

CHAPTER 5

What I and People Who Care about Me Could Do if the 'Tough Time' Happened Again

Congratulations! You've just made a 'Five-Chapter' Story, a hero's story about moving through a 'tough time'. Chapter 1 shows what happened before the 'tough time'. Chapter 2 shows the 'tough time'. Chapter 3 shows what you and others did to help you get through the 'tough time'. Chapter 4 shows a better time later on when things were better and the 'tough time' was over. And Chapter 5 shows what you could do now with help from people who care about you to make sure the 'tough time' doesn't happen again or isn't so bad.

You can make this story into a movie and you can be the director. Like every movie, it helps to add music and movement. Imagine you are the director for your movie. Then, go back and add a drumbeat for each chapter, starting with Chapter 1 and ending with Chapter 5. Next, use a musical instrument such as a xylophone, a keyboard, or a guitar to share your story with music to show how you were feeling. Start with Chapter 1 and make a strong ending for Chapters 4 and 5. Then, just a like a movie director, add action from Chapters 1–5 by showing looks on your face, the loudness and tone of your voice, and what you are doing (movement) in each chapter of your story.[2] The more details you add, the richer your movie will be.

Now, it's time to add some words for your movie. Start by answering the questions below. You can come back later and add more details.

I was _____ years old. This is what happened in Chapter 1, 'Before the "Tough Time"':

_____

_____

_____

_____

_____

_____

_____

This was how I was feeling 'Before the "Tough Time"' on Thermometers.

My Thermometers

Knots (Stress)   Self-control Power   Mad   Sad   Glad   Feel Safe

10 HIGH   10   10   10   10   10   10

1 LOW   1   1   1   1   1   1

This is what happened in Chapter 2, 'The "Tough Time"':

_____

_____

_____

The worst part of the 'tough time' was when

_____

_____

_____

And this was how I was feeling in the worst part of the 'tough time'.

My Thermometers

Knots (Stress)   **Self-control Power**   **Mad**   **Sad**   **Glad**   **Feel Safe**

10 HIGH   10   10   10   10   10   10

1 LOW   1   1   1   1   1   1

Draw how you felt in your body during the worst part of this 'tough time' using different colors for each feeling.

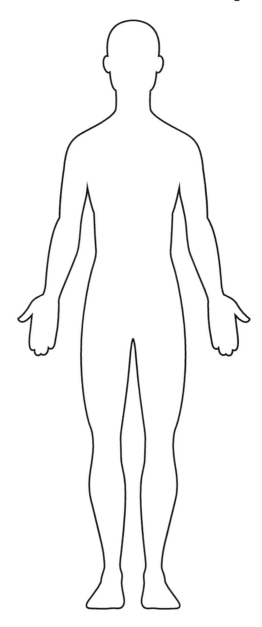

What helped me get through this 'tough time' was that

_____

_____

And, in Chapter 4, when things got better, this is what was happening:

_____

_____

_____

This is how I was feeling when things got better.

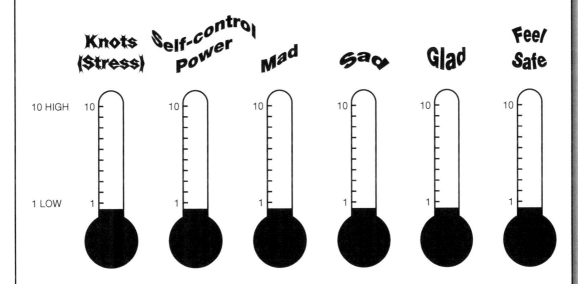

My Thermometers

Most people go through a number of 'tough times'. Sharing them with people you trust can make you stronger.

This is a story of how I got through the next 'tough time' in my life. I am going to draw this story with five pictures that together make a story that begins before the 'tough time' and ends at a time when the 'tough time' was over and I felt safer and better.

[Make your story the same way you did your first Five-Chapter Story.]

[Remember to start on the next page with Chapter 2 of your story. After you draw pictures for Chapters 2, 3, and 4, then draw below what happened before the 'tough time'.]

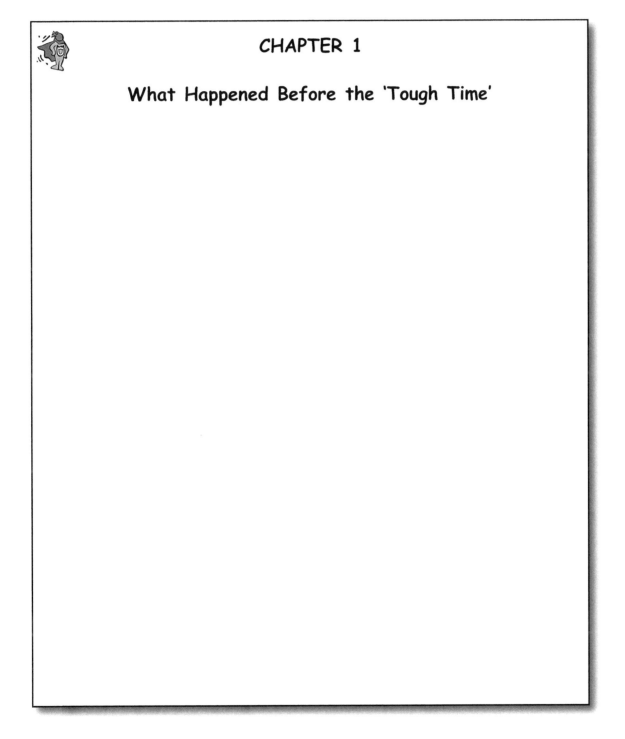

CHAPTER 1

What Happened Before the 'Tough Time'

[Draw what happened in the box below.]

CHAPTER 2

The 'Tough Time'

[Next, show what you and other people did that helped you get through the 'tough time'.]

CHAPTER 3

What Helped Make Things Better

[Next, draw a time when things were better, when you felt safer and the 'tough time' was over. This can be right after the 'tough time', or months or years later.]

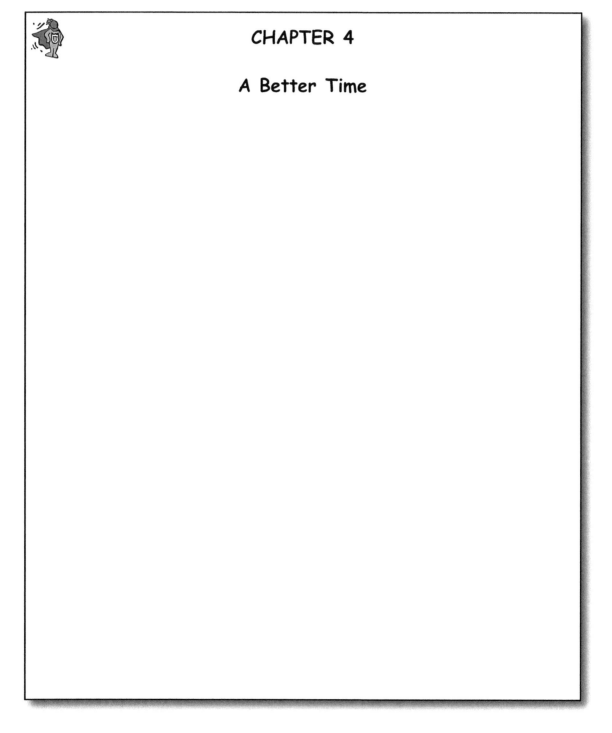

CHAPTER 4

A Better Time

[Go back four pages to draw Chapter 1 of your story, then come back to this page and think about how you are now older, stronger, and smarter. Draw below what you and people who care about you could do to make things better if the 'tough time' started to happen again.]

CHAPTER 5

What I and People Who Care about Me Could Do if the 'Tough Time' Happened Again

Congratulations! You've just made another 'Five-Chapter' Story, a hero's story about moving through a 'tough time'. Imagine you are the director for your movie. Then, go back and add a drumbeat for each chapter. Next, use a musical instrument such as a xylophone, a keyboard, or a guitar to share feelings with music for each chapter of your story. Start with Chapter 1 and make a strong ending with Chapters 4 and 5. Then, show action from Chapters 1–5 with looks on your face, the loudness and tone of your voice, your posture, movement, or show what happened with puppets or a dance. The more details you add, the richer your movie will be.

Now it's time to add some words and feelings for your movie. Start by answering the questions below. You can come back later and add more details to make your movie stronger.

I was _____ years old. This is what happened in Chapter 1, 'Before the "Tough Time"':

_____

_____

_____

_____

_____

_____

_____

This was how I was feeling 'Before the "Tough Time"' on Thermometers.

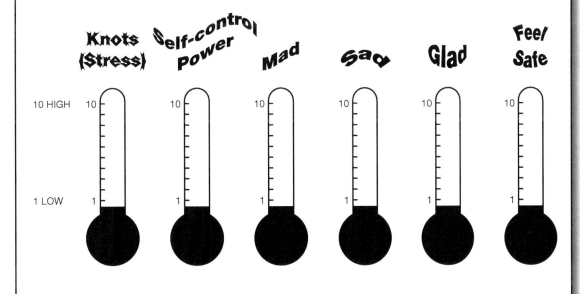

This is what happened in Chapter 2, 'The "Tough Time"':

_____

_____

_____

The worst part of the 'tough time' was when

_____

_____

_____

And this was how I was feeling in the worst part of the 'tough time'.

My Thermometers

Knots (Stress)   **Self-control Power**   **Mad**   **Sad**   **Glad**   **Feel Safe**

10 HIGH   10   10   10   10   10   10

1 LOW   1   1   1   1   1   1

Draw how you felt in your body during the worst part of this 'tough time' using different colors for each feeling.

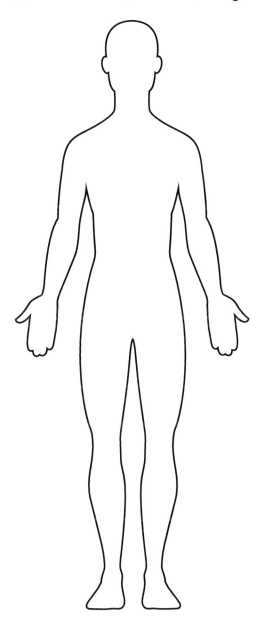

What helped me get through this 'tough time' was that

_____

_____

And, in Chapter 4, when things got better, this is what was happening:

_____

_____

_____

This is how I was feeling when things got better.

My Thermometers

Knots (Stress)	Self-control Power	Mad	Sad	Glad	Feel Safe

10 HIGH

1 LOW

This is a story of how I got through the next 'tough time' in my life. I am going to draw this story with five pictures that together make a story that begins before the 'tough time' and ends at a time when the 'tough time' was over and I felt safer and better.

[Make your story the same way you did your first Five-Chapter Story.]

[Remember to start on the next page with Chapter 2 of your story. After you draw pictures for Chapters 2, 3, and 4, then draw below what happened *before* the 'tough time'.]

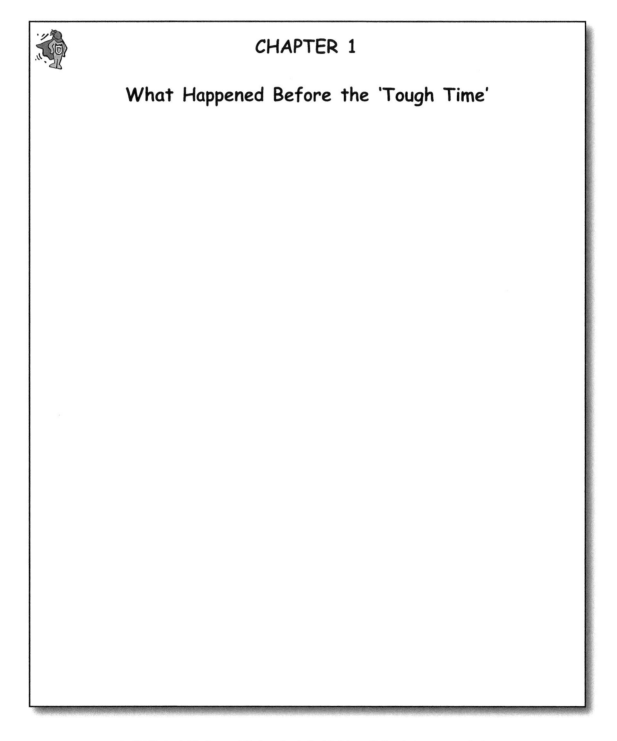

CHAPTER 1

What Happened Before the 'Tough Time'

[Draw what happened in the box below.]

CHAPTER 2

The 'Tough Time'

[Next, show what you and other people did that helped you get through the 'tough time'.]

CHAPTER 3

What Helped Make Things Better

[Next, draw a time when things were better, when you felt safer and the 'tough time' was over. This can be right after the 'tough time', or months or years later.]

CHAPTER 4

A Better Time

[Go back four pages to draw Chapter 1 of your story, then come back to this page and think about how you are now older, stronger, and smarter. Draw below what you and people who care about you could do to make things better if the 'tough time' started to happen again.]

CHAPTER 5

What I and People Who Care about Me Could Do if the 'Tough Time' Happened Again

Congratulations! You've just made another 'Five-Chapter' Story, a hero's story about moving through a 'tough time'. Imagine you are the director for your movie. Then, go back and add a drumbeat for each chapter. Next, use a musical instrument such as a xylophone, a keyboard, or a guitar to share feelings with music for each chapter of your story. Start with Chapter 1 and make a strong ending with Chapters 4 and 5. Then, show action from Chapters 1–5 with looks on your face, the loudness and tone of your voice, your posture, movement, or show what happened with puppets or a dance. The more details you add, the richer your movie will be.

Now it's time to add some words and feelings for your movie. Start by answering the questions below. You can come back later and add more details to make your movie stronger.

I was _____ years old. This is what happened in Chapter 1, 'Before the "Tough Time"':

_____

_____

_____

_____

_____

_____

_____

This was how I was feeling 'Before the "Tough Time"' on Thermometers.

My Thermometers

Knots (Stress)   **Self-control Power**   **Mad**   **Sad**   **Glad**   **Feel Safe**

10 HIGH   10   10   10   10   10   10

1 LOW   1   1   1   1   1   1

This is what happened in Chapter 2, 'The "Tough Time"':

_____

_____

_____

The worst part of the 'tough time' was when

_____

_____

_____

And this was how I was feeling in the worst part of the 'tough time'.

My Thermometers

Knots (Stress)   **Self-control Power**   **Mad**   **Sad**   **Glad**   **Feel Safe**

10 HIGH   10   10   10   10   10   10

1 LOW   1   1   1   1   1   1

Draw how you felt in your body during the worst part of this 'tough time' using different colors for each feeling.

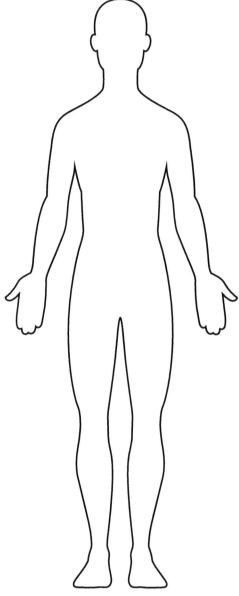

What helped me get through this 'tough time' was that

_____

_____

And, in Chapter 4, when things got better, this is what was happening:

_____

_____

_____

This is how I was feeling when things got better.

My Thermometers

| Knots (Stress) | Self-control Power | Mad | Sad | Glad | Feel Safe |

10 HIGH

1 LOW

This is a story of how I got through the next 'tough time' in my life. I am going to draw this story with five pictures that together make a story that begins before the 'tough time' and ends at a time when the 'tough time' was over and I felt safer and better.

[Make your story the same way you did your first Five-Chapter Story.]

[Remember to start on the next page with Chapter 2 of your story. After you draw pictures for Chapters 2, 3, and 4, then draw below what happened *before* the 'tough time'.]

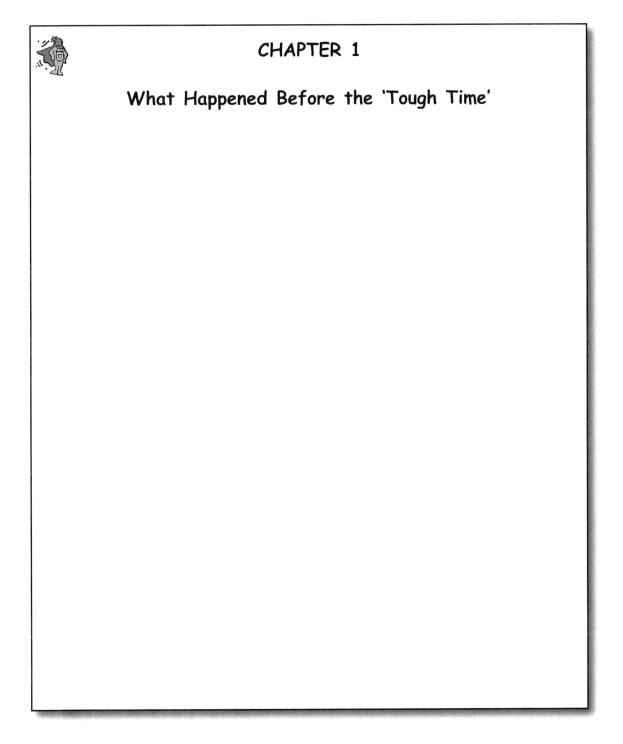

CHAPTER 1

What Happened Before the 'Tough Time'

[Draw what happened in the box below.]

CHAPTER 2

The 'Tough Time'

]Next, show what you and other people did that helped you get through the 'tough time'.]

CHAPTER 3

What Helped Make Things Better

[Next, draw a time when things were better, when you felt safer and the 'tough time' was over. This can be right after the 'tough time', or months or years later.]

CHAPTER 4

A Better Time

Go back four pages to draw Chapter 1 of your story, then come back to this page and think about how you are now older, stronger, and smarter. [Draw below what you and people who care about you could do to make things better if the 'tough time' started to happen again.]

CHAPTER 5

What I and People Who Care about Me Could Do if the 'Tough Time' Happened Again

Congratulations! You've just made another 'Five-Chapter' Story, a hero's story about moving through a 'tough time'. Imagine you are the director for your movie. Then, go back and add a drumbeat for each chapter. Next, use a musical instrument such as a xylophone, a keyboard, or a guitar to share feelings with music for each chapter of your story. Start with Chapter 1 and make a strong ending with Chapters 4 and 5. Then, show action from Chapters 1–5 with looks on your face, the loudness and tone of your voice, your posture, movement, or show what happened with puppets or a dance. The more details you add, the richer your movie will be.

Now it's time to add some words and feelings for your movie. Start by answering the questions below. You can come back later and add more details to make your movie stronger.

I was _____ years old. This is what happened in Chapter 1, 'Before the "Tough Time"':

_____

_____

_____

_____

_____

_____

This was how I was feeling 'Before the "Tough Time"' on Thermometers.

My Thermometers

Knots (Stress) **Self-control Power** **Mad** **Sad** **Glad** **Feel Safe**

10 HIGH

1 LOW

This is what happened in Chapter 2, 'The "Tough Time"':

_____

_____

_____

The worst part of the 'tough time' was when

_____

_____

_____

And this was how I was feeling in the worst part of the 'tough time'.

My Thermometers

Knots (Stress)   Self-control Power   Mad   Sad   Glad   Feel Safe

10 HIGH   10   10   10   10   10   10

1 LOW   1   1   1   1   1   1

Draw how you felt in your body during the worst part of this 'tough time' using different colors for each feeling.

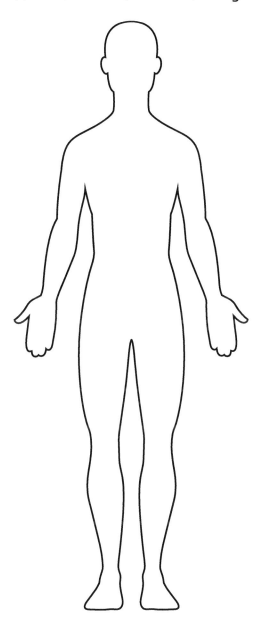

What helped me get through this 'tough time' was that

_____

_____

And, in Chapter 4, when things got better, this is what was happening:

_____

_____

_____

This is how I was feeling when things got better.

My Thermometers

Knots (Stress)	Self-control Power	Mad	Sad	Glad	Feel Safe

10 HIGH   10   10   10   10   10   10

1 LOW   1   1   1   1   1   1

This is a story of how I got through the next 'tough time' in my life. I am going to draw this story with five pictures that together make a story that begins before the 'tough time' and ends at a time when the 'tough time' was over and I felt safer and better.

[Make your story the same way you did your first Five-Chapter Story.]

[Remember to start on the next page with Chapter 2 of your story. After you draw pictures for Chapters 2, 3, and 4, then draw below what happened *before* the 'tough time'.]

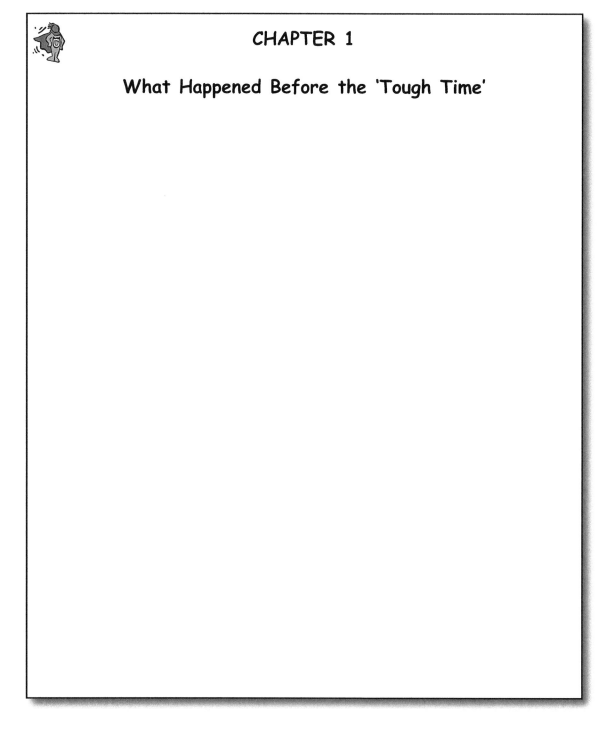

CHAPTER 1

What Happened Before the 'Tough Time'

[Draw what happened in the box below.]

CHAPTER 2

The 'Tough Time'

[Next, show what you and other people did that helped you get through the 'tough time'.]

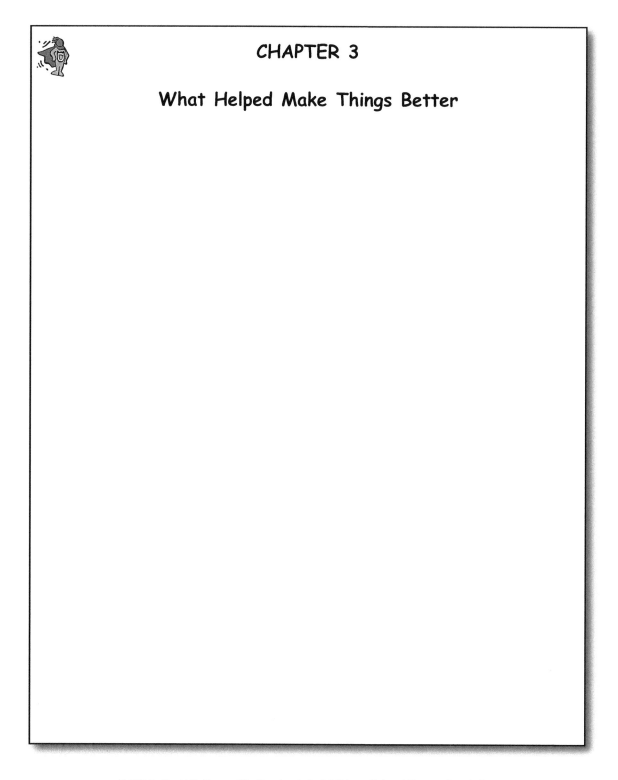

CHAPTER 3

What Helped Make Things Better

[Next, draw a time when things were better, when you felt safer and the 'tough time' was over. This can be right after the 'tough time', or months or years later.]

CHAPTER 4

A Better Time

[Go back four pages to draw Chapter 1 of your story, then come back to this page and think about how you are now older, stronger, and smarter. Draw below what you and people who care about you could do to make things better if the 'tough time' started to happen again.]

CHAPTER 5

What I and People Who Care about Me Could Do if the 'Tough Time' Happened Again

Congratulations! You've just made another 'Five-Chapter' Story, a hero's story about moving through a 'tough time'. Imagine you are the director for your movie. Then, go back and add a drumbeat for each chapter. Next, use a musical instrument such as a xylophone, a keyboard, or a guitar to share feelings with music for each chapter of your story. Start with Chapter 1 and make a strong ending with Chapters 4 and 5. Then, show action from Chapters 1–5 with looks on your face, the loudness and tone of your voice, your posture, movement, or show what happened with puppets or a dance. The more details you add, the richer your movie will be.

Now it's time to add some words and feelings for your movie. Start by answering the questions below. You can come back later and add more details to make your movie stronger.

I was _____ years old. This is what happened in Chapter 1,
'Before the "Tough Time"':

_____

_____

_____

_____

_____

_____

_____

This was how I was feeling 'Before the "Tough Time"' on
Thermometers.

My Thermometers

Knots (Stress)   Self-control Power   Mad   Sad   Glad   Feel Safe

10 HIGH   10   10   10   10   10   10

1 LOW   1   1   1   1   1   1

This is what happened in Chapter 2, 'The "Tough Time"':

_____

_____

_____

The worst part of the 'tough time' was when

_____

_____

_____

And this was how I was feeling in the worst part of the 'tough time'.

My Thermometers

Knots (Stress)   **Self-control Power**   **Mad**   **Sad**   **Glad**   **Feel Safe**

10 HIGH   10   10   10   10   10   10

1 LOW   1   1   1   1   1   1

Draw how you felt in your body during the worst part of this 'tough time' using different colors for each feeling.

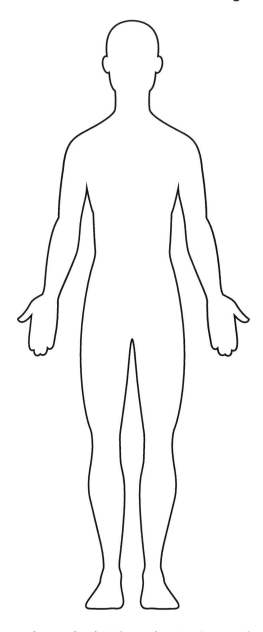

What helped me get through this 'tough time' was that

_____

_____

And, in Chapter 4, when things got better, this is what was happening:

_____

_____

_____

This is how I was feeling when things got better.

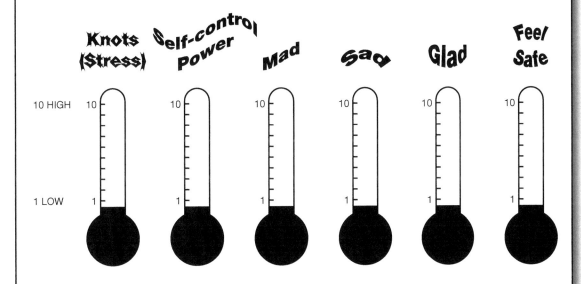

My Thermometers

Knots (Stress)   Self-control Power   Mad   Sad   Glad   Feel Safe

10 HIGH

1 LOW

This is a story of how I got through the next 'tough time' in my life. I am going to draw this story with five pictures that together make a story that begins before the 'tough time' and ends at a time when the 'tough time' was over and I felt safer and better.

[Make your story the same way you did your first Five-Chapter Story.]

[Remember to start on the next page with Chapter 2 of your story. After you draw pictures for Chapters 2, 3, and 4, then draw below what happened *before* the 'tough time'.]

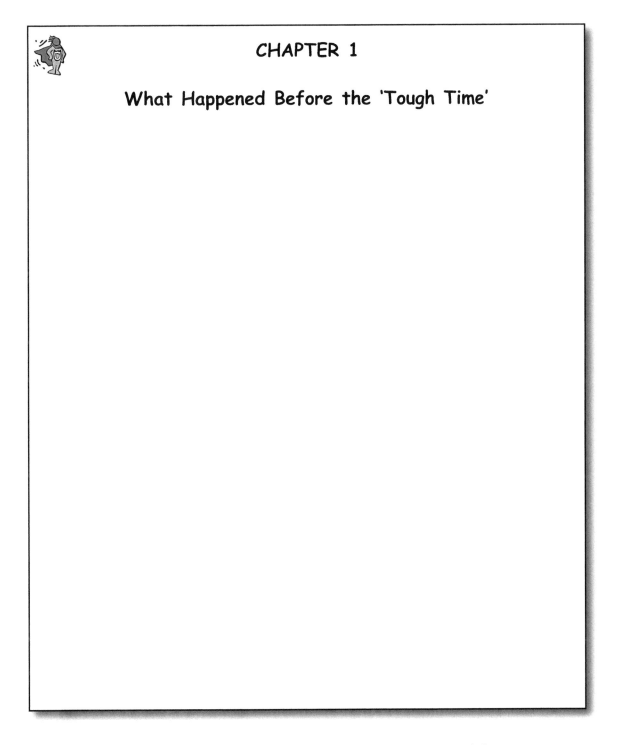

CHAPTER 1

What Happened Before the 'Tough Time'

[Draw what happened in the box below.]

CHAPTER 2

The 'Tough Time'

[Next, show what you and other people did that helped you get through the 'tough time'.]

CHAPTER 3

What Helped Make Things Better

[Next, draw a time when things were better, when you felt safer and the 'tough time' was over. This can be right after the 'tough time', or months or years later.]

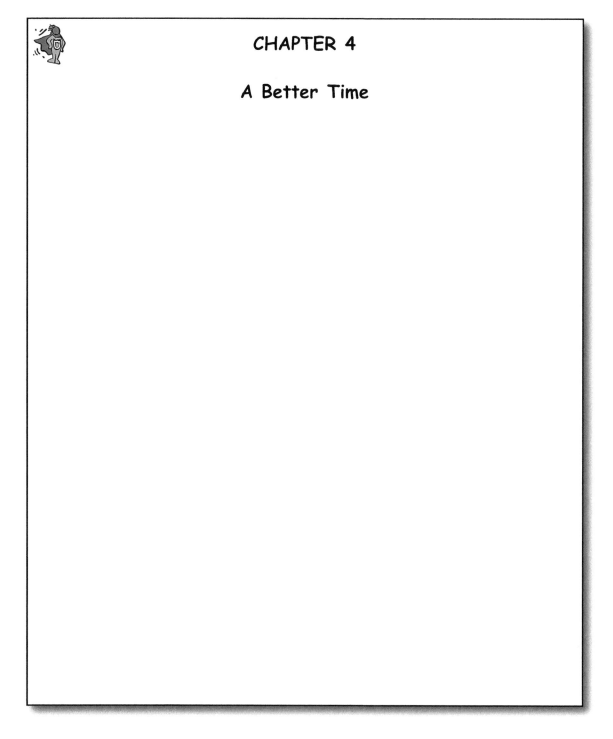

CHAPTER 4

A Better Time

[Go back four pages to draw Chapter 1 of your story, then come back to this page and think about how you are now older, stronger, and smarter. Draw below what you and people who care about you could do to make things better if the 'tough time' started to happen again.]

CHAPTER 5

What I and People Who Care about Me Could Do if the 'Tough Time' Happened Again

Congratulations! You've just made another 'Five-Chapter' Story, a hero's story about moving through a 'tough time'. Imagine you are the director for your movie. Then, go back and add a drumbeat for each chapter. Next, use a musical instrument such as a xylophone, a keyboard, or a guitar to share feelings with music for each chapter of your story. Start with Chapter 1 and make a strong ending with Chapters 4 and 5. Then, show action from Chapters 1–5 with looks on your face, the loudness and tone of your voice, your posture, movement, or show what happened with puppets or a dance. The more details you add, the richer your movie will be.

Now it's time to add some words and feelings for your movie. Start by answering the questions below. You can come back later and add more details to make your movie stronger.

I was _____ years old. This is what happened in Chapter 1, 'Before the "Tough Time"':

_____

_____

_____

_____

_____

_____

This was how I was feeling 'Before the "Tough Time"' on Thermometers.

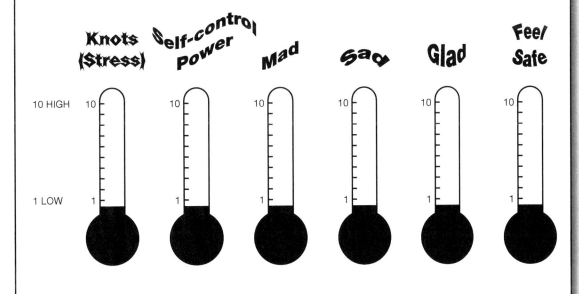

This is what happened in Chapter 2, 'The "Tough Time"':

_____

_____

_____

The worst part of the 'tough time' was when

_____

_____

_____

And this was how I was feeling in the worst part of the 'tough time'.

My Thermometers

Knots (Stress)   Self-control Power   Mad   Sad   Glad   Feel Safe

10 HIGH   10   10   10   10   10   10

1 LOW   1   1   1   1   1   1

Draw how you felt in your body during the worst part using different colors for each feeling.

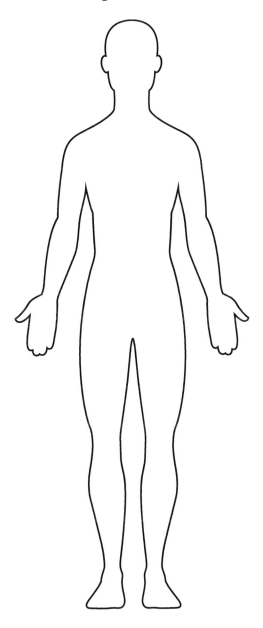

What helped me get through this 'tough time' was that

_____

_____

And, in Chapter 4, when things got better, this is what was happening:

_____

_____

_____

This is how I was feeling when things got better.

My Thermometers

Knots (Stress)	Self-control Power	Mad	Sad	Glad	Feel Safe

10 HIGH

1 LOW

This is a picture (or a photograph) of me when I learned an important lesson about how to make things a little better for myself and the people I care about to get through a 'tough time'.

I was _____ years old. What made it so hard was that

_____

_____

What helped me get through the hard part was

_____

_____

Now that I am older, I know that

_____

_____

This is how I would handle the same thing now. [Draw a second picture of this 'tough time' and add in someone who could help you.]

This is what could help in this picture.

_____

_____

This is what I would look like if you made me into a game card, showing me during the 'toughest' of my 'tough times'.

In this picture, I was _____ years old. The worst part was

_____

_____

What I did was

_____

_____

My power score would be [pick a number between 1 and 100, with
100 being the highest]

_____

My weakness would be

_____

_____

What helped me in this 'toughest' time was

_____

_____

This is what I would look like if I was a hero on a game card and had to
handle the same thing again. [Make up another game card of yourself.]

My powers would include

_____

_____

I would get help from

_____

_____

If I was ever in trouble, I could

_____

_____

[Now imagine yourself growing bigger and bi**gger** with greater abilities to handle problems until you fill the next page.[3] Draw yourself in or have a photograph of yourself enlarged to fill up the page and put your name on the top in large letters.]

People can help each other, but it takes courage. In real life, heroes feel scared. It is easier to run away from trouble than to do something that helps.

If one of my 'tough times' happened to someone I cared about, I would tell them

_____

_____

And, to help them make things better, I would

_____

_____

After I helped someone face a 'tough time', I would feel

_____

_____

And, if someone asked what kind of person I was, I would say I was

_____

_____

We have all done things we regret, everyone, moms and dads, girls and boys, famous athletes and actors, even governors and presidents. Heroes know that there are ways to help make things better when they've done something wrong, even if they did the 'wrong' thing on purpose. It takes courage to say you're sorry and even more courage to help make things better after you've done something that hurt someone.

One thing I'd like to say I was sorry about was

_____

_____

I was _____ years old when this happened. Now that I'm older, I would like to tell _____ that I am sorry for what I did.

If I am ever tempted to make the same mistake again, I am going to remind myself to

_____

_____

And, to help make up for it, I would like to

_____

_____

Another thing I did that hurt someone was to

_____

_____

I was _____ years old when this happened. Now that I'm older, I would like to tell _____ that I am sorry for what I did.

If I am ever tempted to make the same mistake again, I am going to remind myself to

_____

_____

And, to help make up for it, I would like to

_____

_____

[Draw a picture below of yourself making things better.]

Another time I made someone feel bad was when I

_____

_____

I was _____ years old when this happened. Now that I'm older, I would like to tell _____ that I am sorry for what I did.

If I am ever tempted to make the same mistake again, I am going to remind myself to

_____

_____

And, to help make up for it, I would like to

_____

_____

[Draw a picture of yourself making things better.]

The worst mistake I made was probably when I

_____

_____

To help make up for that mistake, and make things better for anyone I hurt, this is what I did, or what I'd like to do.

_____

_____

And, if I am ever tempted to make the same mistake again, I am going to remind myself to

_____

_____

Here's a picture below of me making things better.

Chapter 11

Into the Future

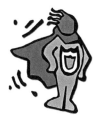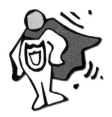

Now that I am _____ years old, I can look back at my life through the happy times, the times when I felt proud, and also the times when I felt sad, scared, lonely, ashamed, or mad. There were good times and bad times. I know that that is true for most people. I also know that I can change what I do the next time I am reminded of good times or bad times. And, I can use what I have learned to help make things better for myself and other people.

I can also look ahead. This is a drawing or a photograph of how I look now.

Looking back, what helped me feel good about myself was

_____

_____

Looking ahead, what I really want to do is

_____

_____

If I were to pick an animal or a picture, similar to a coat of arms, to show how I would like to feel in the future, it would look like [draw it below]

The best part about growing up and becoming older would be that I could

_____

_____

When I am _____ years old, I would like to

_____

_____

If I looked at myself in the mirror, this is what I would notice that I liked about myself at _____ years old.

_____

_____

As a _____-year-old, I could help _____
[This could be a friend, a family member, or an organization in your community that helps people.]

This is what I could do to help

_____

_____

Here is a drawing of what I would look like helping someone when I am a few years older, when I am _____ years old.

This is a picture of how I will look when I am 28 years old. I would like to be working as a _____

The best part about growing up and becoming an adult would be that I could

_____

_____

Someday, I would like to be a _____ and help people by

_____

_____

If I looked at myself in the mirror, this is what I would notice that I liked about myself

_____

_____

If I had a bumper sticker on my car, it would say

When I am grown up, I would like to share my most special times with

_____

_____

[Draw a picture of how you would share a special time and who you would share it with.]

When I turn 40 years old, I would like to celebrate my birthday by

_____

_____

[Draw a picture of how you would like to celebrate and who you would like to have with you. Or, if you would rather, draw a T-shirt that you could wear after your party and write a message on it for everyone to see.]

The best part of my celebration would be when

_____

_____

Chapter 12

My Story

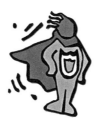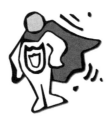

When I think about all the pictures and stories in this book, I think that the most important thing that I did to make things better was to

_____

_____

If I met a boy or a girl who was living the way I used to live when I was going through 'tough times', this is what I could tell that boy or girl to help him or her feel better.

_____

_____

And then, I could tell that boy or girl an important lesson that I learned in my life about what helps you to get through 'tough times' and make things better.

_____

_____

MY LIFE STORY

[Please use the next pages to write a story about your life from the time you were born, a story that shares the most important things that happened and how you grew stronger, smarter, and braver with help from people who cared about you. Write about what made the good times 'good' and how you learned to get through the 'tough times'. Please also include pictures or photographs of important people. You can also make your story into a movie for you to keep and share with people you trust.]

[Please read the Heroes Creed below and then write what you think makes a person a real life hero.]

HEROES CREED

It takes action to free ourselves from living in fear.

Action requires energy to move.

We can get energy by using our fears. Everyone has fears. We feel fear in our bodies. Fears warn us to be ready. Fears can energize us to move. We can use fear as energy to move forwards or lose ourselves in the grip of our fears. Accepting and using our fears makes us stronger.

Action also requires courage.

The secret to courage is purpose. It means finding out what you need to do to make things better. And, it means believing with all your heart that something you can do can make a difference.

But action alone does not make a real hero.

Action for heroes means doing something to make things better and doing it together with other people who help each other.

Action for heroes means helping others and getting help for ourselves.

Congratulations!

You finished your *Life Storybook*!

You can make your own cover by using the blank space on page 21 of the *Life Storybook*.

Before you go, please write a message on the next pages to share some of the lessons you learned about what helps to become 'stronger and stronger' and get through 'tough times'. That's one way that heroes help other people. This could be a message to help other children who may have 'tough times' of their own. You can also add a dedication page to honor special people in your life.

What I learned about getting through the 'tough times'

_____

_____

_____

_____

_____

_____

_____

_____

_____

_____

_____

_____

_____

_____

_____

_____

_____

_____

THIS BOOK IS DEDICATED TO

_____

_____

Certificate of Completion

By completing the

Real Life Heroes Life Storybook,

_____

has shown the courage to remember

the past, to make the most of the present,

and to build a better future.

_____

_____

_____

[Signatures of adult witnesses]

_____

[Date]

Notes

CHAPTER 1: THE HEROES CHALLENGE

1. Ford, J. D. (2005) Trauma Treatment Implications of Altered Affect Regulation and Information Processing Following Child Maltreatment. *Psychiatric Annals*, 35(5): 410–419.
2. Sutton, P. (2003) Personal communication.
3. Adapted from Ford, J. D. & Russo, E. (2006). A Trauma-Focused, Present-Centered, Emotional Self-Regulation Approach to Integrated Treatment for Post-Traumatic Stress and Addiction: Trauma Adaptive Recovery Group Education and Therapy (TARGET). *American Journal of Psychotherapy*, 60(4): 335–355.
4. Ibid.
5. Ibid.
6. This card can be laminated or made into a magnet.
7. Adapted from Ford, J. D. & Russo, E. (2006). A Trauma-Focused, Present-Centered, Emotional Self-Regulation Approach to Integrated Treatment for Post-Traumatic Stress and Addiction: Trauma Adaptive Recovery Group Education and Therapy (TARGET). American Journal of Psychotherapy, 60(4): 335–355.
8. Mahoney, K., Ford, J. D., & Cruz St. Juste, M. C. (2005) *TARGET-A: Trauma Adaptive Recovery Group Education and Therapy (10+ Session Adolescent Version) Facilitator Guide*. Farmington, CT: University of Connecticut Health Center.

CHAPTER 2: A LITTLE ABOUT ME

1. This figure is from www.bing.com, licensed under Creative Commons.
2. Instructions on this page and next adapted from Ford, J. D. & Russo, E. (2006). A Trauma-Focused, Present-Centered, Emotional Self-Regulation Approach to Integrated Treatment for Post-Traumatic Stress and Addiction: Trauma Adaptive Recovery Group Education and Therapy (TARGET). *American Journal of Psychotherapy*, 60(4): 335–355.

CHAPTER 4: POWER PLANS

1. *A Caregiver's Power Plan* is available in *Real Life Heroes Toolkit for Treating Traumatic Stress in Children and Families* (Routledge).
2. Checklists below adapted from Foster Family Programs of Hawaii FFP Respite/School Tool.
3. Adapted from TARGET -Worksheets. Ford, J. D. & Russo, E. (2006). A Trauma-Focused, Present-Centered, Emotional Self-Regulation Approach to Integrated Treatment for Post-Traumatic Stress andAddiction: Trauma Adaptive Recovery Group Education and Therapy (TARGET). *American Journal of Psychotherapy*, 60(4): 335–355.
4. Adapted from Foster Family Programs of Hawaii FFP Respite/School Tool.

CHAPTER 6: IMPORTANT PEOPLE

1. Adapted from M.D. Evans (1986) *This Is Me and My Two Families*. New York: Magination Press.

CHAPTER 7: MIND POWER

1. Adapted from Goleman, D. (2014). Cited by Ruth Buczynski, PhD Concentration and the Brain—Training Your Brain for Better Focus. January 31, 2014. National Institute for the Clinical Application of Behavioral Medicine. www.nicabm.com/nicabmblog/concentration-and-the-brain/.
2. Ibid.
3. Children should be able to calm themselves enough to stay in control before moving ahead to Chapter 10. Use of thermometers as outlined in the *Real Life Heroes Toolkit* can help therapists determine if a child is sufficiently stable to work on trauma desensitization with support from safe caregivers. If necessary, therapists and caregivers can practice different ways for children to calm down or find someone who can help them feel more safe and comfortable before moving on. Please see the *Real Life Heroes Toolkit* for guidelines, skill-building activities, and strategies to help children and caregivers become able to manage their stress well enough to work on Chapter 10.

CHAPTER 8: CHANGING THE STORY

1. Adapted from Marra, T. (2004). *Depressed & Anxious: The Dialectical Behavior Therapy Workbook for Overcoming Depression & Anxiety*. Oakland, CA: New Harbinger Publications.
2. All images of the figure on this page are from www.bing.com licensed under Creative Commons.
3. Adapted from Ford, J. D. & Russo, E. (2006). A Trauma-Focused, Present-Centered, Emotional Self-Regulation Approach to Integrated Treatment for Post-Traumatic Stress and Addiction: Trauma Adaptive Recovery Group Education and Therapy (TARGET). *American Journal of Psychotherapy*, 60(4): 335–355.
4. Adapted from Marra, T. (2004). *Depressed & Anxious: The Dialectical Behavior Therapy Workbook for Overcoming Depression & Anxiety*. Oakland, CA: New Harbinger Publications.
5. Adapted from Siegel, D. J. (2014). *Brainstorm: The Power and the Purpose of the Teenage Brain*. New York: Penguin.

CHAPTER 9: LOOKING BACK

1. Thanks to Suzanne d'Aversa for recommending this section.

CHAPTER 10: THROUGH THE 'TOUGH TIMES'

1. Chapter 10 should be guided by a licensed therapist trained in trauma treatment following safety criteria provided in *Real Life Heroes Toolkit for Treating Traumatic Stress in Children and Families*.
2. You can also show what happened with puppets or a dance.

3. Adapted from Ramon Rojano (1998) Community Family Therapy, Workshop presented at the Sidney Albert Fall Institute, Albany, New York, October 9.